John Haygarth, FRS

(1740–1827)

A Physician of the Enlightenment

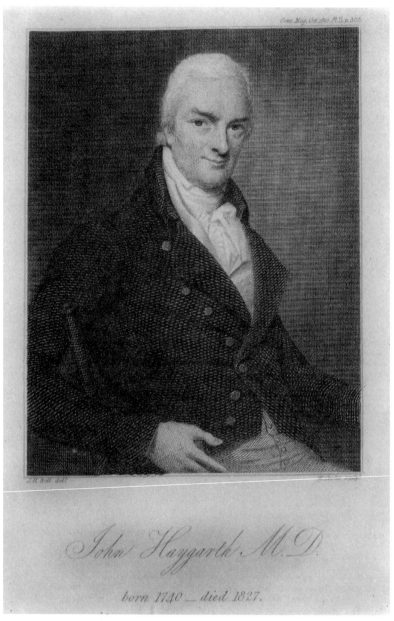

John Hygarth M.D.

born 1740 — died 1827.

John Haygarth
(Courtesy of the Wellcome Library, London)

John Haygarth, FRS

(1740–1827)

A Physician of the Enlightenment

CHRISTOPHER BOOTH

*The Wellcome Trust Center for the
History of Medicine
at
University College London*

AMERICAN PHILOSOPHICAL SOCIETY
PHILADELPHIA•2005

Memoirs
of the
American Philosophical Society
Held at Philadelphia
For Promoting Useful Knowledge
Volume 254

ISBN: 0-87169-254-6
US ISSN: 0065-9738

Library of Congress Cataloging-in-Publication Data

Booth, Christopher C. (Christopher Charles), 1924–
    John Haygarth, FRS (1740–1827) : a physician of the enlightenment / Christopher Booth.
        p. ; cm. — (Memoirs of the American Philosophical Society held at Philadelphia for
    promoting useful knowledge, ISSN 0065-9738 ; v. 254)
    Includes bibliographical references and index.
    ISBN-13: 978-0-87169-254-2 (cloth)
    ISBN-10: 0-87169-254-6 (cloth)
        1. Haygarth, John, 1740–1827. 2. Physicians—England—Biography.   I. Title. II. Memoirs
    of the American Philosophical Society ; v. 254.
        [DNLM: 1. Haygarth, John, 1740–1827.   2. Physicians—Great Britain—Biography. 3.
    Clinical Medicine—history—Great Britain. WZ 100 H421B 2005]
    Q11.P612 vol. 254
    [R489.H35]
    081 s–dc22
    [610.92 B]
                                            2005045285

To my grandchildren

Contents

Contents

Preface

Let us preserve the memory of the deserving:
perhaps it may prompt others likewise to deserve

John Fothergill, letter to Dr William Cuming, Dec 8, 1769[1]

*T*he century of the Enlightenment was a remarkable era of British History. It was not, as in France, dominated by an elect group of *Philosophes.* Certainly, John Locke's *Essay on the Human Understanding* and Newton's *Principia Mathematica* were its literary touchstones. But as an intellectual movement, the Enlightenment in England owed much to clubs, societies, and coffee-houses where men debated the issues of the day, often in a hot and smoky environment.[2] There they perused a press freed from censorship and enjoyed the prints of cartoonists who were merciless in their portrayals of the high and mighty. They could also read the new novelists who sought to describe the foibles of the contemporary world, whilst Boswell recorded the conversations and opinions of his hero, Dr. Johnson. It was, furthermore, an era when philanthropy increasingly established its importance in the national life.

During that century the Industrial Revolution in England transformed society and Britain established its imperial role. Despite the implacable opposition of the monarch, the first modern republic was founded by British colonists in America. At the same time, the remaining unknown areas of the habitable world were explored. After James Cook returned from his circumnavigation of the world in the *Endeavour,* the first print of a kangaroo was published in London and at the instigation of Sir Joseph Banks, who had travelled with Cook, the earliest settlements in Australia were established.

In such a century it is not surprising that medical men should have made material contributions to progress. John Locke's great contribution

[1] J. C. Lettsom. *The Works of John Fothergill MD.* London, Charles Dilly, 1784.

ix

had been to define in philosophical terms the scientific outlook of Newton. Himself a physician, he regarded Boyle, Newton and his close friend Thomas Sydenham as the master builders of knowledge, and saw himself as an underlabourer who cleared the ground a little and removed the rubbish that lay in the way of knowledge. Samuel Johnson too, writing in the introduction to the first edition of his *Dictionary* described himself as "the slave of science . . . doomed only to remove rubbish and clear obstructions from the path of learning and genius. . . ."[3] But for the medicine of his time, Johnson's definition of the word "Physick" was significant. He echoed Locke who had written: "Was it my business to understand Physick, would not the safe way be to consult nature herself in the history of diseases and their cures rather than espouse the principles of the dogmatists. . . ." In fact, it was during the eighteenth century that the practice of medicine came to be regarded as a science. Johnson himself, in that first edition, defined "Physick" as the "science of healing."[4]

There was during the century of the Enlightenment a progressive rejection of "the principles of the dogmatists." Galen had dominated medical thought since the time of the Romans. Now, stimulated in Britain by Newtonian science and organisations such as the Royal Society, whose motto was *Nullius in verba,* observation and experiment came to replace the empty theorising that had formed the basis of medical thought for so long. Yet there have been many who have derided the medicine of that era, remembering today only the excessive purgation and bleeding to which the afflicted were subjected. Furthermore, the eighteenth century has been seen by some historians as a fallow period sandwiched between two centuries of scientific achievement—the seventeenth dominated by William Harvey and his followers and the nineteenth by the emergence of the bacterial origins of human disease, cellular pathology, natural selection and the discoveries of William Röntgen. This notion has had support from distinguished scientists. In the 1930s a President of the Royal Society went so far as to express the view that there had been no outstanding advance in the theory and practice of medicine during the entire eighteenth century and he quoted William

[2] Roy Porter. *Enlightenment.* London, Allen Lane, The Penguin Press, 2000.

[3] Samuel Johnson. *A Dictionary of the English Language.* London; Knapton, Longman, Hitch and Hawes, Millar and Didsley, 1755.

[4] See also: Christopher C Booth. Clinical science in the Age of Reason. *Perspectives in Biology and Medicine* 1981–2; 25: 93–114.

Osler, physician, bibliophile, and scholar, who had written: "What a vast literature exists between Sydenham and Broussais. What a desolate sea of theory and speculation."[5] It is remarkable that a century which witnessed the conquest of scurvy amongst seamen, the discovery of digitalis (still in use today), the introduction of vaccination (which has now conquered smallpox throughout the world), and the description of both the nature of oxygen and the anaesthetic properties of nitrous oxide should have been so unceremoniously consigned to the dustbin of history.

In fact the eighteenth century was an era when Enlightenment men, among them physicians who had studied either at Leiden under Herman Boerhaave or at the Medical School at Edinburgh, sought in many ways to improve the lot of their fellow citizens. Some, for example William Heberden, are remembered for the disorders they described, others, like William Withering, for treatments that they introduced. John Hunter, an unlettered surgeon, became one of the leading biologists of his age, his legacy at the Royal College of Surgeons in London being his museum. There were also those like John Hunter's pupil, Edward Jenner, who sought to prevent disease, his discovery of vaccination proving to be the most important of the entire eighteenth century. Yet there were many other individuals, such as the provincial physician and polymath, Erasmus Darwin of Lichfield, whose lives, often unsung, were equally devoted to the improvement of the practice of medicine. John Haygarth of Chester and Bath was one of these. The measures that he proposed for the prevention of infectious fevers were as important as many of the discoveries of his eighteenth-century colleagues. He was also, like his Quaker contemporaries John Fothergill and John Coakley Lettsom, devoted to philanthropic ideals. He sought with some success to improve the schooling of the children of the poor and was a pioneer in the development of Savings Banks in England. Yet he has been neglected by historians, perhaps because, as John Haygarth himself pointed out, his work, although novel, excited little controversy at the time. Haygarth was a figure of considerable significance in the medical Enlightenment of the eighteenth century in England. That is why he deserves to be remembered today.

[5] F. Gowland Hopkins. Anniversary address. *Proc R Soc B,* 1934; 114:181–205.

Acknowledgments

$\mathcal{J}$ wish to acknowledge the help of many people who have contributed to this biographical study of John Haygarth. I am particularly indebted to Whitfield J. Bell of the American Philosophical Society for his work on the Edinburgh Medical School during the eighteenth century and for allowing me to quote from his biographical memoir of Arthur Lee. Stella Miller-Collett, professor of classical and Near Eastern archaeology at Bryn Mawr College, was very helpful in providing details of the Haygarth family, particularly those concerning William Haygarth, the doctor's elder son. I also thank W. F. Bynum for his help and advice on the problems of fever in the eighteenth century and for drawing my attention to Haygarth's correspondence with William Cullen. In addition, I am grateful to Roger Rolls of the Bath and Wessex Medical History Group for information on the social scene in Bath in John Haygarth's time and for explaining the different scientific and philosophical societies that existed in Bath. He was also kind enough to read the manuscript.

I acknowledge with thanks the help of Olive Haygarth with details of Dr. Haygarth's forbears; Elspeth Griffiths, archivist at the library of Sedbergh School, for her searches of the registers of Sedbergh School and for contributing John Haygarth's letter to John Harrison; Denise Colton, who generously allowed me access to the Badgerdub Papers in her possession, in particular the doctor's account books and his correspondence with his nephew, James Haygarth; Joyce Scobie and other members of the Sedbergh and District Historical Society, who were most helpful in responding to queries; Jonathan Harrison of the library of St. John's College, Cambridge, who provided important information on Cambridge University in the eighteenth century, particularly with reference to the teaching of medicine; the librarian of the Edinburgh University Library for details of John Haygarth's matriculation records; the permanent secretary of the Royal Medical Society on Haygarth's election to the society; the library of the University of Virginia for providing copies of the letters of Arthur Lee when a student in Edinburgh to his brother Richard Henry Lee; Katy Goodrum of the Cheshire Record Office for material relating to Haygarth's home in Chester and information on the early years of the Chester Royal Infirmary; the library of the Royal Society for the details of John Haygarth's nomination and election to the fellowship of the society; the librarian of the Manchester Literary and Philosophical Society; R.H.T. Edwards for information on the Brocken spectre; T. J. Peters for drawing my attention to Dr. Haygarth's interest in canal schemes; Richard J. Wolfe of the Francis A. Countway Library of Medicine at Harvard University for the details of Haygarth's honorary degrees; Margaret DeLacy for information on influenza in eighteenth-century Britain; the Warwick County Record Office for John Haygarth's letter to Thomas Pennant; the Mitchell Library, Sydney, New South Wales, for permission to reproduce the letter to Sir Joseph Banks; Jane Coates of the Bath Royal Literary and Scientific Institution; the Bath City Library; T. H. Spencer Tizzard, onetime owner of No. 15, The Royal Crescent, for information from the title deeds of his property; the librarian of the Temple Reading Room, Rugby School; the Kendal Record Office; and Gabriel Linehan of the Lambeth Palace Library for responding to many queries.

The librarians of the Royal College of Physicians of London, the Wellcome Library for the History and Understanding of Medicine, and the library of the College of Physicians of Philadelphia have kindly permitted me to quote from letters from their collections.

I would also like to express my particular thanks to Christopher Lawrence of the Wellcome Centre for the History of Medicine at University College, London, for reading the manuscript and for making many valuable suggestions. Professor Harold Cook and Dr. E. M. Tansey have provided valuable support.

Finally, I thank Maria Karkucinski of Book Design Studio and Mary McDonald of the American Philosophical Society for their work ensuring the book's publication.

List of Illustrations

xv

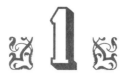

Health Care in the England of John Haygarth

*J*ohn Haygarth (1740–1827), physician to the infirmary in the northern English town of Chester, was an Enlightenment man. Typical of his age, he was generous and philanthropic, amiable yet determined, with interests that ranged from the prevention of infectious fevers and the control of smallpox to the provision of church schools and the management of savings banks. Unlike many of his dissenting friends and contemporaries, he was a committed Anglican. He sought, like so many of his provincial contemporaries, to improve the lot of his fellow men. Men such as Haygarth should not be dismissed as "mere provincials," for during the eighteenth century it was provincials in England who made some of the major contributions to the medicine of their day. The conquest of scurvy following Lind's work with the Royal Navy, the discovery of oxygen by Joseph Priestley, the introduction of digitalis by William Withering of Birmingham, the study of nitrous oxide by Humphry Davy in Bristol, and the demonstration by Edward Jenner in his native Gloucestershire of the efficacy of vaccination against smallpox were all achievements which were made by "provincials."

John Haygarth's contribution was of similar importance, yet it was so simple and in retrospect so self-evident that it has not had the recognition that it deserves. He showed, for the first time, how isolation procedures could prevent the spread of common infectious fevers and how the removal of patients with fever from their homes to special wards in hospitals, where they could receive care, could stop epidemics. He was a pioneer in his concern for the public health. It was Haygarth's work that led to the establishment of fever hospitals in nineteenth-century Britain.[1]

[1] Biographical studies of John Haygarth include John Elliott, "A Medical Pioneer: John Haygarth of Chester," *British Medical Journal* 1 (1913): 235–242; George H. Weaver, "John Haygarth: Clinician, Statistician, Investigator, Apostle of Sanitation," *Bulletin of the Society*

The Social Background

For most of his life John Haygarth lived in a century characterized by "the overthrow of absolutism, accelerating population growth, urbanisation, a commercial revolution marked by rising disposable income, [and] the origins of industrialisation."[2] It was also a century during which, throughout the land, laudable attempts were made to bring whatever benefits contemporary health care might offer to the less fortunate in society.

Many medical men contributed to this endeavor. Some were bewigged and ornate physicians, fellows of the Royal College in London. There were others, however, who were dissenters, barred from the upper echelons of the medical establishment because they were not graduates of the two English Universities, which also refused them entry. Many others, like Haygarth, pursued their careers in English country towns, where they became significant figures in local society and were able freely to indulge their interests and to encourage philanthropy among their fellow citizens. In whatever stations they held, however, none were able to escape the social changes that surrounded them and influenced their lives so greatly.

The rise in population in England was perhaps the social change that had the most immediate impact. It was most marked in the second half of the century: there were just over six million inhabitants of England in 1700, only half a million more in 1750, but by 1811 the population was over ten million. In London, where one-tenth of the population lived, the population tripled from 300,000 in 1700 to more than 900,000 by the turn of the century. Throughout the land the pattern was the same, particularly in those towns where the effect of increasing industrialization was most marked. Manchester was a relatively small borough in the middle of the century, with a population of as little as 17,000. By the early nineteenth century it numbered 180,000 souls. Chester, where Haygarth lived for nearly thirty years, had by his time yielded its position as an ancient port to nearby Liverpool. For this reason, the population of Chester, by contrast with surrounding

of Medical History Chicago 4 (1930): 156–200. Particularly on Haygarth and smallpox, see a prize-winning essay, Francis M. Lobo, "John Haygarth, smallpox and religious dissent in eighteenth century England," in *The Medical Enlightenment of the Eighteenth Century,* ed. Andrew Cunningham and Roger French (Cambridge: Cambridge University Press, 1990), 217–253. See also A. W. Downie, "John Haygarth of Chester and Inoculation against Smallpox," *Liverpool Medical Institution Transactions and Report for the Year 1964* (Liverpool, Medical Institution Library, 1964), 26–42.

[2] Roy Porter, *Enlightenment* (London: Penguin Press, 2000), 12.

cities, showed no great population increase. Haygarth's estimate of the population of Chester in 1774 was 14,713 and at the time of the 1801 census it had only reached 15,052.[3] Working in a relatively small population may well have been an advantage to Haygarth. Unlike many of his contemporaries in the metropolis or in the expanding towns of the Industrial Revolution, he was able to persuade his fellow citizens to courses of action that could not be pursued so readily elsewhere.

In London, as in other cities, there was a great increase in the number of inhabitants. It was the pressure of population that forced them to leave the old city and congregate in the outer parishes beyond its ancient confines. The wealthy moved to the west, upwind of a metropolis that stank with the excrement of a variety of domestic animals as well as the stench that arose from open drains and sewers. Future householders in the west of the city were also persuaded that they would get first use of the waters of the River Thames. This was a period when so many of the elegant Georgian squares were built in west London. Bloomsbury was increasingly popular among the well-to-do. Dr. John Fothergill, the Quaker physician and philanthropist who was a role model to John Haygarth and his contemporaries, moved from Gracechurch Street in the city to Harpur Street, Bloomsbury, in 1767. There, in the words of a visitor in 1770, the street was "perfectly still and quite unlike the idea I had formed of the hustle and bustle of London."[4]

This tranquil environment in which the well-to-do lived was in striking contrast to the dwellings of the lower classes, who increasingly pressed eastward, inhabiting rickety tenements that often fell down, as well as basements and garrets that teemed with families often living in unbelievable squalor. Fires were frequent, with a high mortality rate. The endless courts and unkempt streets provided an ideal environment for the many petty crooks and worse sheltering there, as well as encouraging the spread of disease, particularly infectious fevers. London physician John Coakley Lettsom, fellow Quaker and protégé of John Fothergill and correspondent of John Haygarth, pointed out of the poor in general that these unfortunates "by successive attacks of illness . . . are incapable of procuring the common necessities of life; they have literally wanted bread, as well as cloaths, and instead of a bed I have often seen an oilcloth substituted, and the whole furniture has been a worn-out blanket, insufficient to hide what decency requires. On such a

---

[3] Information from Cheshire Record Office, Chester.

[4] Christopher C. Booth, "Ann Fothergill: The Mistress of Harpur Street," *Proceedings of the American Philosophical Society* 122 (1978): 340–354.

couch I have often found a husband, a wife, one, two, or three children at once chained by disease, without any resources to procure a morsel of bread."[5] The next step might be worse, for they might be sent to Newgate as debtors, many being unable to pay the exorbitant rents of landlords, or more often landladies. For the nation's physicians, there was no question in those times of the link between poverty and ill health.

The situation was as bad if not worse in many towns throughout the land. In Whiggish Manchester, physicians like Thomas Percival and John Ferrier, both dissidents but friends of John Haygarth in the nearby Tory town of Chester, were deeply concerned with the conditions of the laboring poor. Most had migrated to the town in search of work in what became, during the second half of the eighteenth century, "the site of the world's first large industrial society."[6] By then Manchester was the center of the growing textile trade. Percival was a pioneer in pressing for factory legislation. Many cotton mills were totally insanitary, encouraging the propagation of fevers. They were injurious to the constitutions of those who worked in them, with deficient ventilation leading to hot and impure air. The custom of keeping the machines working twenty-four hours, throughout the day and night, was particularly responsible for deficient ventilation, and all doors and windows were blocked during periods of cold weather. Children were undoubtedly the greatest sufferers.

Liverpool was the major port for importing the raw materials that Manchester required. By the 1770s the American cotton trade produced as much as five million pounds by weight annually. At the same time, traffic in slaves was one of the major activities of Liverpool merchants and shipmasters. The population of the city was swollen by the influx of workers in the expanding mercantile industries, as well as poor immigrants, particularly from Ireland, who flooded in to find work. James Currie, who came to share John Haygarth's concern with the frequent epidemics of fever that afflicted the poor, arrived in Liverpool in 1780. Like Lettsom, he was frankly horrified by the obvious effect on the public health of poor housing, insanitary practices, and overcrowding. Currie roundly condemned unregulated lodging houses as well as "the unhealthiness of the cellar dwellings [where thousands lived in the depths of squalor] and the pernicious practice of building the new labourers houses in small confined courts which have a communication

[5] Christopher Booth, "1773," *Transactions of the Medical Society of London* 114 (1998–1999): 79–91.

[6] John V. Pickstone, *Medicine and Industrial Society* (Manchester: Manchester University Press, 1975).

with the street by a narrow aperture but no passage of air through them, and without drainage or cleansing, and greatly overcrowded."[7] It was an intolerable situation that did not receive attention in Liverpool until the next century, when W. H. Duncan, the first medical officer of health in the country, a nephew of Dr. Currie, persuaded the borough to take radical steps through legislation to improve the living conditions and health of the laboring poor.

Development of New Medical Institutions

In both London and the provinces it became clear that medical facilities, particularly for the poor, were either totally inadequate or entirely absent. The Poor Law was increasingly unable to provide for the needs of the homeless and the destitute. It was a period when neither governments nor local authorities saw the provision of health care as their problem. As Smollett cogently put it, "No Mycaenas appeared among the ministries and not the least patronage glimmered from the throne."[8] Nothing was more needed than philanthropy, so that the prosperous could lend aid to the poor and disadvantaged. Fortunately, the increasing prosperity of the capital and of provincial towns meant that many men and women of substance in society wished to make contributions. But, as Donna Andrew has argued, it would be wrong to consider the institutions created by philanthropy as only concerned with the improvement of the physical health of the population. There was often a religious motive as well.[9] When St. George's Hospital was founded in 1733, it was thought that it would lead to "an increase of True Religion and Piety among the Common People." Thomas Coram (1668–1751) had similar thoughts in his mind when he established the Foundling Hospital in 1739, which was to be devoted to the "preservation as well as the education of abandoned and illegitimate children." The many lying-in hospitals in London founded at that time and the Lock Hospital for venereal diseases shared the same ideals.

In fact, medical philanthropy was to develop in two different but complementary ways. During the first half of the century it was the foundation of

[7] R. D. Thornton, *James Currie, The Entire Stranger and Robert Burns* (Edinburgh and London: Oliver and Boyd, 1963).

[8] F. M. L. Poynter, *The Evolution of Hospitals in Britain.* (London: Pitman Medical Publishing Company, Ltd., 1864), 60.

[9] Donna T. Andrew, *Philanthropy and Police: London Charity in the 18ᵗʰ Century* (Princeton: Princeton University Press, 1989). See also Dorothy Marshall, *The English Poor in the 18ᵗʰ Century* (London: George Routledge and Sons, 1926).

new hospitals that captured the imagination of contemporary philanthropists. In London, hospitals were established to augment the three ancient monastic foundations available to London's citizens at the beginning of the century: St. Bartholomew's, St. Thomas's, and the hospital for the mentally afflicted at Bethlem. Five new "voluntary" hospitals were founded in that era—Westminster Hospital (1720), Guy's Hospital (1724), St. George's Hospital (1733), the London Hospital (1740), and the Middlesex Hospital (1745). They were funded by well-meaning citizens and supported by private subscribers, who were able to recommend patients in proportion to their subscriptions.[10]

By the later decades of the century, however, it had become apparent that the hospitals alone could not cope with the increasing health needs of the population. Furthermore, the hospitals, fearful of importing infection, excluded cases of fever, one of the most common illnesses in those crowded and unhygienic times. The appearance in the last quarter of the eighteenth century of the "Dispensary Movement" was, according to Loudon, due to "the manifest failure of the hospitals to evolve, adapt and enlarge to meet the crisis in health care at the end of the century."[11] At the end of the seventeenth century a short-lived dispensary was run by the College of Physicians in London, but the eighteenth-century dispensary was in fact John Coakley Lettsom's brainchild. The dispensary for poor children founded by George Armstrong in Red Lion Square in 1769 may well have influenced Lettsom. During the winter of that year the young physician frequently crossed Red Lion Square to make visits to the home of John Fothergill in Harpur Street. He was at the time conducting a flirtation with Dr. Fothergill's niece Betty, who was visiting from her home in Warrington.

Lettsom founded the general dispensary at Aldersgate in London in 1770; he was not yet 26 years old. Deeply concerned for the tribulations of the poor, he wrote, "The poor are a large, as well as useful part of the community; they supply both the necessary and ornamental articles of life; and they have, therefore, a just claim to the protection of the rich."[12] The object of the dispensary

---

[10] Poynter, *The Evolution of Hospitals in Britain*. See also John Woodward, *To Do the Sick No Harm: A Study of the British Voluntary Hospital System to 1875.* (London: Routledge and Kegan Paul, 1974).

[11] I. S. L. Loudon, "The Origins and Growth of the Dispensary Movement in England," *Bulletin of the History of Medicine* 55 1981: 22–42. See also R. Kirkpatrick, "'Living in the Light': Dispensaries, Philanthropy and Medical Reform in Late Eighteenth Century London," in *The Medical Enlightenment of the Eighteenth Century,* ed. Andrew Cunningham and Roger French (Cambridge: Cambridge University Press, 1990), 254–280. It is likely that Lettsom's mentor, John Fothergill, may have taken a sympathetic interest in the Aldersgate Dispensary, for its first president was the Earl of Dartmouth, half-brother to Lord North and a patient of Fothergill.

was not only to provide health care to the poor as outpatients at the dispensary, but also to encourage visits by the staff of the dispensary to the sick and afflicted poor in their own homes, an entirely new enterprise. The risk to their lives was real and ever present. Lettsom was to lose a valued and much-loved son to a fever contracted through his dispensary work. Fever was to become a major concern for John Haygarth, but in Chester there was no dispensary. Instead, Haygarth in the infirmary in Chester successfully pioneered receiving wards to which cases of fever were freely admitted.

In London, dispensary subscribers were sought in the same way that hospital supporters were recruited. For the Aldersgate Dispensary the subscription was one guinea a year, permitting the recommendation of one patient. The success of the Aldersgate Dispensary was never in doubt. The number of subscribers rose from 100 in 1770 to 600 in 1773, and to 1,400 by 1778. Soon dispensaries were springing up all over the capital, so that by the end of the century there were fourteen.

In many provincial towns the care of the sick and destitute had been undertaken by ancient monastic or church foundations that dated from medieval times. As in London, however, they could not deal with the health problems of their increasing populations. They followed the example of the capital. The earliest provincial voluntary hospitals were founded in Winchester (1736) and Bristol (1737). Other towns soon followed suit. During the 1740s seven more were established (York, Exeter, Bath, Northampton, Worcester, Shrewsbury, and Liverpool), and by the end of the century there were twenty-eight provincial hospitals throughout the land. The Chester Infirmary, whose staff Haygarth joined in 1767, was founded in 1753. Of the towns where the satanic mills of the Industrial Revolution emerged, Manchester founded its infirmary as early as 1752, but Birmingham only followed in 1773 and the Sheffield Infirmary was not established until 1797.[13]

[12] J. C. Lettsom, *Medical Memoirs of the General Dispensary in London for the Years 1773–74* (London: E. and C. Dilly, 1774). See also Christopher Booth, "1773." The Aldersgate Dispensary was not the first to be founded in London. If one ignores the short-lived dispensary set up by the Royal College of Physicians at the end of the seventeenth century, that honor should go to George Armstrong, who established the Dispensary for the Infant Poor in Red Lion Square in 1769.

[13] For examples of the history of provincial hospitals in England, see William Brockbank, *Portrait of a Hospital: 1752–1948* (London: William Heineman, 1952); S. T. Anning, *The General Infirmary at Leeds: The First Hundred Years 1767–1869* (Edinburgh and London: E. & S. Livingstone, 1963); John Thackeray Bunce, *A History of the Birmingham General Hospital* (Birmingham: Messrs. Cornish Brothers, 1873). See also Stanley Barnes, *The Birmingham Hospital Centre* (Birmingham: Stanford and Mann, 1952).

At the same time, dispensaries were spreading to the provinces. An aspiring physician might begin with dispensary work. When James Currie went to Liverpool in 1780, his first appointment was to the dispensary; only later was he to become one of the physicians at the Liverpool Infirmary.

Emergence of Professional Staff for the New Hospitals

It is remarkable that during those years there was an adequate number of medical men to staff the newly developing hospitals and dispensaries in England. Rather by chance than by design, it was the University of Leiden in the early decades of the century and the Edinburgh Medical School later that had the most influence in training young men. At Edinburgh not all took a medical degree, many either opting for attending classes or going elsewhere to graduate, as did John Haygarth. The two ancient universities at Oxford and Cambridge insisted on seven years of study and a master's degree before the undergraduate could begin to study medicine. It took as long as fourteen years to obtain an MD. Therefore, as Dr. Johnson advised a young American, Arthur Lee from Virginia, who was considering a career in medicine,

> If you have a large Fortune, & time enough to spare, go to either of these. (But) if you would choose immediately to enter upon Physic, and to attain sufficient knowledge therein, to carry you through Life, & at a small Expense, & in a short time, by all means (go) to Edinburg or Leyden; for the Scotch or foreign Education is like a House built to last a man's lifetime only; The English is like a Palace, or fortress intended to last for many Ages. The first build slightly, the last lay a very strong and firm Foundation before they begin the Work.[14]

Perhaps the great lexicographer was influenced by the views of his own much admired physician and classical scholar, William Heberden, his "ultimus Romanorum," who had both graduated from and for a while taught at Cambridge. However firm Johnson may have considered the foundation for a medical career that was available at the two English universities, they were quite unable to provide the increasing number of medical men who were required to staff the new medical institutions throughout the land, nor could their numbers in any way keep pace with the health care needs of

---

[14]Whitfield J. Bell. "Arthur Lee (1740–1792)," in *Patriot Improvers: Biographical Sketches of Members of the American Philosophical Society,* vol. 3 (Philadelphia: American Philosophical Society, in press).

the expanding urban populations. Furthermore, there were many, including the Edinburgh-trained physician John Fothergill, who were contemptuous of the English universities of that era. Fothergill wrote to the keeper of the Ashmolean Museum in 1769,

> I do not know of anything that would give me more pain than to reside a few months at Oxford. I should discover men of the first rate of understanding, partly from want of experience, partly from want of opportunity, but more from indolence, absorbed in an insignificant round of doing that which the lowest of mankind enjoy as much as themselves: eating, drinking and sleeping.[15]

Fothergill's comments recall those of Edward Gibbon (1737–1794), who was admitted to Magdalen College, Oxford, in 1752 at the age of 15. He wrote in later years that the months he spent at Oxford were the most idle and unprofitable of his whole life. It was a period when the university was plunged in port and prejudice.

Leiden's claim to be an important center for medical education had been established long before the emergence of Herman Boerhaave, whose lectures to students of medicine started in 1701. During his lifetime, Boerhaave held a position as a medical teacher that was unrivalled in Europe, and he had a major impact in providing the medical graduates who were to staff the new hospitals in England.[16] Between 1701 and his death 37 years later, 746 English-speaking students matriculated in the medical faculty of Leiden University.[17] The subsequent careers of Boerhaave's English students (345 of the total) show that in England in the early eighteenth century the educated elite of Leiden graduates played a key role in shaping the future of medicine in England, particularly as physicians to the newly founded voluntary hospitals in both the capital and the provinces. The first physician to the Westminster Hospital was Alexander Stewart, fellow of the Royal Society, Copley medalist, and MD of Leiden in 1711. Guy's Hospital appointed its first two physicians when it was founded in 1725—John Oldfield and James Jurin, both Leiden graduates. When St. George's Hospital opened its doors in 1733, five men who had been

---

[15] Betsy C. Corner and Christopher C. Booth, *Chain of Friendship: Selected Letters of Dr. John Fothergill of London 1735–1780* (Cambridge: Bellknap Press of Harvard University Press, 1971), 300.

[16] Christopher Booth, "Herman Boerhaave and the British," *Journal of the Royal College of Physicians of London* 23 1989: 129–197.

[17] R. W. Innes-Smith, *English-Speaking Students at the University of Leiden* (London and Edinburgh: Oliver and Poyd, 1932).

pupils of Hermann Boerhaave were appointed to posts as physicians in the first eighteen months. There was no lack of applications for positions in the voluntary hospitals, since by taking on this work for no remuneration a physician might greatly increase his status in society.

In the many English provincial hospitals founded during the eighteenth century the story was the same. At Bristol, for example, the colorful William Logan had been a pupil of Boerhaave, and at the York County Hospital, founded in 1740, four of the early physicians were Boerhaave's men. They included the man-midwife John Burton, the original for Dr. Slop in Sterne's *Tristram Shandy*. At Bath, William Oliver, inventor of the Bath Oliver biscuit and friend of Alexander Pope and Richard Nash, had been a student at Leiden in 1720. Even ecclesiastic preferment may have been influenced by Boerhaave, for Thomas Secker, MD of Leiden in 1721, became Archbishop of Canterbury in 1758. It was not unusual for men of the cloth to involve themselves closely with the voluntary hospital movement; the Rev. Alured Clarke, prebend of the cathedral, not only played a major role in founding the first provincial hospital at Winchester, but after his translation to the deanship of Exeter he also led the movement for the establishment of the Devon and Exeter Hospital in 1741. Archbishop Secker himself warmly applauded the efforts of these pioneers.[18]

After the death of Boerhaave in 1738, Edinburgh inherited the position that had been Leiden's for so long. The Edinburgh Medical School was founded by Alexander Monro (primus) (1697–1767).[19] In 1726 he was joined by four men who had all been students of Boerhaave in Leiden and who now sought to establish medical teaching on the Leiden model in the Scottish capital: Alexander Rutherford (1695–1779),[20] Andrew St. Clair (1697–1760), Andrew Plummer (1698–1756), and John Innes (1696–1733).[21] In the later years of the century a Glasgow graduate translated to Edinburgh, William Cullen (1710–1790) became, like Boerhaave, the most acclaimed teacher of his time.[22]

[18]Woodward, *To Do the Sick No Harm.*

[19]Alexander Monro (1697–1767), in *Oxford Dictionary of National Biography* (hereafter *Oxford DNB*) (H. C. G. Matthew and Brian Harrison, Eds.: Oxford, The University Press, 2004), 38:638–640.

[20]Alexander Rutherford (1695–1779), *Oxford DNB;* 48:389–390. Rutherford was Sir Walter Scott's maternal grandfather.

[21]Douglas Guthrie, *The Medical School of Edinburgh* (Edinburgh: George Waterston and Sons, 1959).

[22]William Cullen M. D. (1710–1790), *Oxford DNB;* 14:581–586.

The influence of Edinburgh graduates on medicine in England was soon felt. John Fothergill was a Quaker barred from the English universities because of his beliefs. He graduated from Edinburgh in 1736 and was the first Edinburgh graduate to become a licentiate of the Royal College of Physicians in London. Having no degree from Oxford or Cambridge, he was barred from ever becoming a fellow, but he went on to achieve a practice in the capital that was second only to that of Dr. Johnson's admired physician, William Heberden.[23] Within the new voluntary hospitals throughout England, the presence of Edinburgh graduates was increasingly apparent. Although in both Oxford and Cambridge the physicians to the new hospitals (Addenbroooke's in Cambridge and the Radcliffe at Oxford) were graduates of the university who happened to be local practitioners, the Manchester Infirmary appointed Samuel Kay, MD of Edinburgh, as a physician when it was founded in 1752. When the Leeds General Infirmary opened its doors in 1767, the five first physicians were all Edinburgh men, as were three of the foundation physicians at the Birmingham General Hospital in 1773, although John Ash, considered the founder of the hospital, was an Oxford graduate. At both Liverpool and Chester, Edinburgh men were to be preeminent.

John Haygarth was to become a Cambridge MB, but it was undoubtedly the teaching he received in Edinburgh that most shaped his ideas. How Haygarth, a young lad from an isolated valley of North Yorkshire, went from his position in a provincial hospital to become a distinguished physician and medical philosopher, with a fellowship of the Royal Society and an international reputation, illustrates the career opportunities available to ambitious men of the eighteenth century.

---

[23] Ernest Heberden, *William Heberden: Physician of the Age of Reason* (London: Royal Society of Medicine Services, 1989).

Upbringing and Education

The Haygarths of Garsdale

*J*ohn Haygarth, the future physician in both Chester and Bath, was born at Swarthgill, a manor house in Garsdale, in 1740, the son of William Haygarth.[24] His native dale is a narrow isolated valley that runs westward from its origin in the upper Pennines to the market town of Sedbergh at its foot. Coursed by the tumbling waters of the river Clough, its steep sides make for rugged farming. Haygarth's grandfather, after whom he was named, had moved to Garsdale from his family home in the neighboring valley of Dentdale at the end of the first decade of the eighteenth century. He settled at Swarthgill, where the porch bears a date stone inscribed "I H I 1712," for himself, John Haygarth, and his wife, Isabell Nelson. There are ancient mullioned windows and within there is old oak paneling, similar to that found nearby in other houses of the same period. There are also two spice cupboards, set into the walls, that bear the same inscription as the porch.

[24] Olive Haygarth, "The Haygarths of Dent and Garsdale," *The Sedbergh Historian* 3 (1995): 25–29. John Haygarth was only one of a remarkable group of physicians who in the eighteenth century hailed from that rural area of northwest Yorkshire. William Hillary (1697–1763), author of an important work, *The Diseases of the West India Islands*, and the famous Quaker physician John Fothergill (1712–1780) both came from nearby Wensleydale. Anthony Askew (1722–1772), registrar of the Royal College of Physicians and founder of a famous library, was educated at Sedbergh School, as was Anthony Fothergill (no relation of Dr. John), who was born in Ravenstonedale. Robert Willan (1757–1812), pioneer dermatologist, came from Marthwaite near Sedbergh, and George Birkbeck (1776–1841), also a Quaker, founder of Mechanics Institutes, came from Settle in Ribblesdale. It was there that J. C. Lettsom (1744–1815) served his apprenticeship to the Quaker apothecary, Abraham Sutcliffe. C. C. Booth, "Doctors from the Yorkshire Dales," *Proceedings of the 23rd International Congress of the History of Medicine* (London: Wellcome Institute of the History of Medicine, 1972), 998–1001.

It is difficult to know why the Haygarths, as well as their friends the Inmans of nearby Low House, who migrated from Horton-in-Ribblesdale in 1719, came to such an isolated valley. Perhaps it was the haunting beauty of the place, evident to this day, with its grey stone walls, rushing streams of clear water, and the sunlight and shadow on its tree clad hillsides. Neither family were themselves farmers. The Inmans were well-off gentry and John Haygarth Sr., when he was living in Dent, was involved in the knitting business. In 1712, when he first moved to Swarthgill, he was described as a "hosier." Like other hosiers in the district, such as Robert Willan of Castehow near Sedbergh,[25] he would have made his fortune by acting as a middleman between the local population, whose prowess as knitters of stockings was legendary, and the merchants of Cheapside who sought their wares.[26] The inventories of their wills indicate their relative wealth. It seems likely that John Haygarth used the proceeds of his business as a hosier to purchase property in Garsdale. He continued to be described as a hosier in property deals in 1715–1716 and in 1718. Thereafter he was known as a "yeoman," suggesting that he later gave up his involvement with the knitting trade.[27]

The Inmans were perhaps more intellectually inclined than the Haygarths, for many Inmans, both then and in later generations, went to the local grammar school at Sedbergh and on to Cambridge.[28] The best known was James Inman (1776–1859), who was the senior wrangler at Cambridge in 1800 and later became principal of the Royal Naval College at Portsmouth. Inman's nautical tables were to remain in use for more than forty years. By contrast, John Haygarth, the future physician, was the only member of his family to be educated at Sedbergh School and at Cambridge, his relatives being more committed to rural pursuits. Like the Inmans, however, they were among the members of the Sedbergh Book Club, a forum for the rural intellectuals of those days, which was originally founded in 1728.[29]

[25] C. C. Booth, "The Willans of Marthwaite," *Medical History* 25 (1981): 25–29.

[26] Marie Hartley and Joan Ingilby, *The Old Hand-Knitters of the Dales* (Clapham: Dalesman Publishing Company, 1951).

[27] Bonds and deeds relating to Swarthgill in lower Garsdale, records of the Sedbergh and District History Society.

[28] B. Wilson, *The Sedbergh School Register 1546 – 1909* (Leeds: Richard Jackson, 1909).

[29] C. G. Hollett, "The Story of the Sedbergh Book Club," *Sedbergh and District History Society Newsletter* 5 (1986): 24–30. See also K. A. Manley, "Rural Reading in North-west England: The Sedbergh Book Club 1728–1928," *Book History* 2 (1999): 78–268.

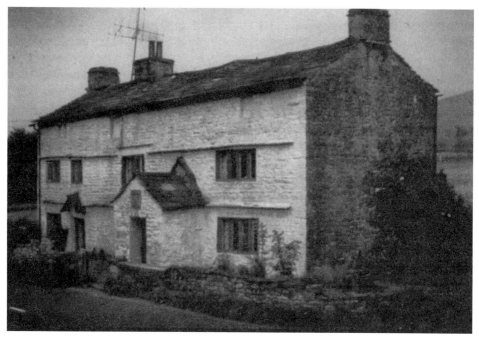

FIG. 1. Swarthgill in Garsdale
(*Photograph by the author.*)

John Haygarth seems to have been a particular favorite of his grandfather. His father William's first wife, Magdalen Metcalfe, whom he married in 1737, sadly died within a few days of the birth of her only son. One can speculate that her death may have been due to puerperal fever. It is likely that the young John Haygarth was brought up by his grandparents at Swarthgill. In 1748, when John was 8 years old, his father married Elizabeth Wray, by whom he had three sons and four daughters. In that same year William Haygarth moved with his new wife to New House, later to be known as Badgerdub, a property owned by his father. It was only a short distance from Swarthgill on the road to Sedbergh. At that time John may well have stayed with his grandparents at the family home, for when old John Haygarth died in 1757 at the age of 82, he left three properties in Garsdale to his grandson, as well as some silver.[30] At this time John's father William inherited New House. John Haygarth Jr. was the only grandchild so favorably treated by the venerable one-time hosier, perhaps indicating the high regard that he had for him.

[30]Will of John Haygarth, Lancashire Record Office.

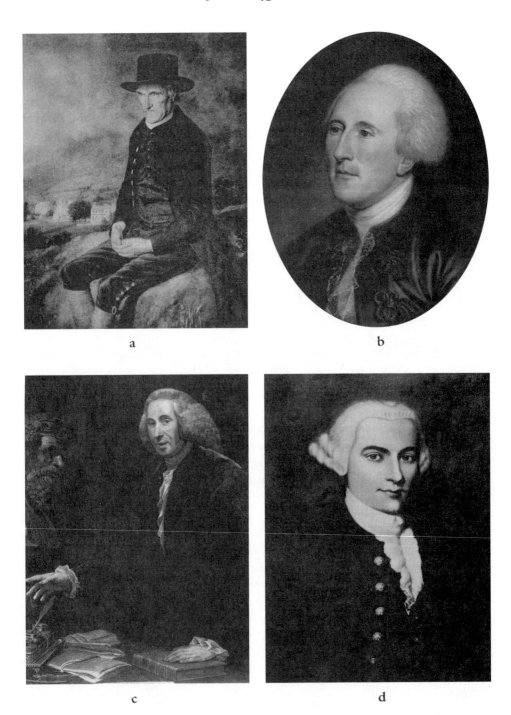

a

b

c

d

Sedbergh School and Haygarth's Mathematical Tutor

The people of Sedbergh and its surrounding district were fortunate in their local grammar school.[31] It is generally thought to have been Roger Lupton, a provost of Eton, who founded the school in 1525. Almost immediately a close link was established with St. John's College, Cambridge, which appointed the master. At the same time, six scholarships were available exclusively for Sedbergh boys after 1527. When in the 1540s many chantries were dissolved by Henry VIII, Sedbergh was saved by St. John's College and by an impassioned sermon from its master, Dr. Lever, before the king, claiming that the school "was most needed in the North Country amongst the rude people in knowledge." For the next three and a half centuries the school continued as a local grammar school, with varying degrees of success. When Posthumous Wharton was headmaster between 1674 and 1706, the number of scholars rose as high as 120. His successor, however, Thomas Dwyer, only attracted 12 boys in the three years of his office. By the time John Haygarth attended the school in the 1750s, Wynne Bateman was the master. He was known for his energy and the force of his character. He was "highly skilled as a classical teacher and equally successful as a teacher of mathematics." The successes of Sedbergh boys in both subjects made the school particularly famous at Cambridge. How effective Bateman was at maintaining discipline, however, is uncertain. People were said "to have made free with him. He has twice been pulled by the nose," wrote a contemporary, "besides being very rudely treated in other ways."[32] Haygarth would have studied in the new school building, built in 1716 in the time of Samuel Saunders as master, the father-in-law of Wynne Bateman.[33] The contact with St. John's College was

---

[31] H. L. Clarke and W. N. Weech, *History of Sedbergh School, 1525–1925.* (Sedbergh: Jackson and Co., 1925).

[32] C. C. Booth, "John Dawson (1734–1820)," *British Medical Journal* 4 (1970): 171–173.

[33] The building is preserved to this day as the school library.

FIG. 2a. John Dawson, with Sedbergh School in the background
(Courtesy of the Wellcome Library, London.)
　　　　b. Arthur Lee
(Courtesy of the National Park Service, Independence National Historical Park.)
　　　　c. William Cullen;
　　　　d. Thomas Percival *(Both courtesy of the Wellcome Library, London.)*

maintained, the master being appointed by the college and specific scholarships being available for selected boys. The school remained a local grammar school until 1874, when control passed from St. John's College to an independent board of governors. Thus was the English Public School of today established, serving well-to-do families in the north of England and taking only a few day boys from the local district.

There is little doubt that Haygarth received an excellent classical education under Wynne Bateman. He was also fortunate in his mathematical tutor, John Dawson.[34] Dawson was born at Raygill Farm, a mile or two up the valley of Garsdale from the Haygarth home at Swarthgill. It was a simple home, his father being a "statesman" who earned little more than 10 or 12 pounds a year. Until he was over 20 years of age, John Dawson worked as a shepherd in the hills. High above Raygill there is a stone called Dawson's rock where, according to local tradition, young Dawson sat and worked out a system of conic sections entirely by himself. His family's limited resources made formal education unavailable to him and according to one account Dawson taught himself by begging or borrowing books and doing a little teaching. As early as 1756, however, when he was 22 years old, his reputation as a rural intellect began to be known locally, and in the summer of that year three young men intending to enter Cambridge went to read with him. The first was the 16-year-old John Haygarth, who thus early in his life developed the mathematical skills that were to be of such significance in his later work, as well as ensuring the friendship of a remarkable individual who would help him throughout his career. The second was Richard Sedgwick, who later became the vicar of Dent and the father of Adam Sedgwick, Woodwardian Professor of Geology at the University of Cambridge. The third was to become an obscure clergyman in Leicestershire. Adam Sedgwick later recalled how his father always spoke of this Garsdale summer with Dawson as one of "great happiness and profit."[35]

Soon after, Dawson became an assistant to Mr. Bracken of Lancaster, a well-known country surgeon and apothecary with a wide and extensive practice. Dawson, too old to be a regular apprentice, learned the rudiments of the profession that was to be his livelihood. Later he set up in practice in Sedbergh. At first he lived a life of extreme abstemiousness, but by the end of his first year had scraped together enough money to finance a journey to

---

[34] Booth, "John Dawson."

[35] Adam Sedgwick. *Supplement to the Memorial to the Trustees of Cowgil Chapel.* Cambridge: Cambridge University Press, 1870.

Edinburgh, where he attended medical classes until his money ran out. Two years later he had saved enough for a visit to London, traveling part of the way by stage wagon, the mode of transport of the poor. London, however, was more expensive than Edinburgh. Furthermore, his mathematical abilities were increasingly recognized and he was unable to lead the unobtrusive life he had followed in the Scottish capital. Returning to Sedbergh, Dawson became a much sought after mathematical tutor, taking students during the summer vacations and after giving up his practice in 1790 devoting himself wholly to mathematical teaching. He charged five shillings a week for instruction and would teach for as long as his pupils wanted to learn. They came from far and wide. Dr. Butler, later headmaster of Harrow, was his pupil in 1792. In a letter he describes his journey from the south and how he paid 1 shilling and 6 pence a week for an excellent room at the best hotel in town, the King's Arms. Breakfast was 2 pence, and dinner could be "a leg of mutton and potatoes both hot; ham and tongue, gooseberry tarts, cheese, butter and bread; pretty well for ten pence."[36]

Between 1781 and 1794 Dawson had seven senior wranglers among his pupils, and the senior wranglers for 1797, 1798, 1800, and 1807 all studied with Dawson. One of these was the Garsdale boy and neighbor of the Haygarths, James Inman, of nautical tables fame.[37] Other Dawson alumni included the Quaker Robert Willan, a Sedbergh boy and Edinburgh graduate who became a well-respected physician in London, founding the specialty of dermatology. Adam Sedgwick and George Birkbeck, the founder of mechanics institutes, were also pupils of Dawson. Whether Dawson was ever himself on the staff of Sedbergh School is uncertain. His links with the school must, however, have been close, for his marriage to Ann Thirnbeck in 1767 was solemnized by John Haygarth's headmaster, Dr. Bateman. In fact, only three of his senior wranglers were Sedbergh men. Haygarth himself was never a wrangler, but his mathematical friendship with his Garsdale neighbor was to stand him in good stead in his later years as a physician.

Dawson published relatively little but he engaged in learned controversy with William Emerson on the question of a slip made by Newton on the problem of precession. In 1769 he published a tract attacking Matthew Stewart, professor of mathematics at the University of Edinburgh, on his

---

[36] "Letter dated Sedbergh 11 June 1792," *The Sedberghian* 28 (1907): 79–80.

[37] Michael Jackson, "James Inman: A Brief Sketch of His Life," *Sedbergh and District History Society Newsletter* 2 (1984): 19–21.

calculations of the distance of the sun from the earth.[38] He pointed out that this could only be done by observing the transit of Venus, the task undertaken by James Cook and his scientific colleagues in Tahiti a year later during his circumnavigation of the globe in the *Endeavour*.

Cambridge

It seems unlikely that John Haygarth would have decided on a medical career during his time at Sedbergh School. Others from the school, seeking to train themselves for a life in medicine, first served apprenticeships to apothecaries for some years before going on to Edinburgh for their university education. John Fothergill had left Sedbergh in 1728 to serve as an apprentice with his fellow Quaker, Benjamin Bartlett of Bradford, going on to Edinburgh in 1734.[39] Anthony Fothergill from Ravenstonedale, namesake but no relation to Dr. John Fothergill, was almost a contemporary of John Haygarth. After his schooling at Sedbergh, he was apprenticed in 1755 to John Drake Bainbridge, an influential figure in Durham, serving for five years before matriculating at Edinburgh.[40] If he was contemplating a medical career, this might well have been an appropriate course for the young Haygarth to follow. In fact, like others of his colleagues who did not study medicine, he went on to St. John's College, Cambridge, in June 1759. There, on June 25, having been examined and approved by Mr. Bateman, he was admitted as pensioner, with Dr. Powell as his tutor.[41] He was also a Hebblethwaite scholar, a position reserved for Sedbergh boys. He may perhaps have felt somewhat overawed on arriving, a country boy, in the city of Cambridge, for his Garsdale friend, Thomas Inman, had graduated in the previous year as the fifth wrangler in the Cambridge Mathematical Tripos, but had died soon afterward. Nevertheless, there was at least one other Sedbergh friend to sustain him. John Hutton of Westmorland, future wrangler, was admitted by Dr. Powell five days after young Haygarth's admission.

[38] J. Dawson, *Pamphlet on Four Propositions,* (Newcastle: J. White and T. Saint, 1769).

[39] R. Hingston Fox, *Dr John Fothergill and His Friends: Chapters in Eighteenth Century Life,* (London: Macmillan, 1919).

[40] Christopher Lawrence, Paul Lucier, and Christopher C. Booth, *"Take Time by the Forelock": The Letters of Anthony Fothergill to James Woodforde, 1789–1813,* Medical History Supplement, no. 17 (London: Wellcome Institute for the History of Medicine, 1997).

[41] Information kindly provided by Jonathan Harrison, special collections librarian, the Library of St. John's College, Cambridge.

The undergraduates of John Haygarth's time would have studied mathematics, classics, philosophy, and theology. William Samuel Powell was a distinguished scholar who was to become senior fellow of his college in 1760 and master in 1765.[42] The subjects that he encouraged give some idea of what Haygarth would have studied during his three years at Cambridge. In the first year, the first book of Horace, the ninth book of the *Iliad*, algebra, and logic; in the second, the first six books of Euclid, the first volume of Locke's *Essays*, and the first two books of Livy; and in the third, hydrostatics and optics, the second book of Grotius *De jure belli et pacis*, and Xenophon on the Lacedaemonian and Athenian Commonwealth.[43] Powell was also insistent on the study of the gospels and in later years, after examinations were introduced by him, all years were also examined on St. Mark's Gospel. Under the influence of Newtonian philosophy, mathematics gradually became the leading study in the university. The Mathematical Tripos was introduced in 1748 and was the only route to an honors degree until 1824, when the Classical Tripos began.

It seems unlikely that John Haygarth learned much at Cambridge of significance to his medical education. For medicine, the eighteenth century was the least satisfactory period of the university's history. In 1840, Peacock wrote,

> The corruption which has characterised and disgraced the government of the last century, and which has filled the colleges with fellows, who were neither distinguished by learning nor high principle, exerted a paralysing influence upon those who might otherwise have been disposed or able to restore the fallen studies and degraded character of the Universities.[44]

In Haygarth's time the Regius Professor of Physic, Russell Plumptre, seems not to have lectured, though his colleague in anatomy, Charles Collignon, gave a course of twenty-eight lectures in the Lent term only. In 1770, Collignon was described by William Cole as the most suitable person for his professorial duties, "as he is a perfect skeleton himself, absolutely a walking skeleton."[45]

[42] William S. Powell (1717–1775), *Oxford DNB;* 45:126–127.

[43] Information from Jonathan Harrison.

[44] Sir Humphrey Davy Rolleston, *The Cambridge Medical School: A Biographical History* (Cambridge: Cambridge University Press, 1932), 14.

[45] Paul Searby, *A History of the University of Cambridge,* vol. 3 (Cambridge: Cambridge University Press, 1992), 193–203. See also Christopher Wordsworth, *Scholae Academicae: Some Account of the Studies at the English Universities in the Eighteenth Century* (Cambridge: Cambridge University Press, 1877), 171–181.

There is, however, no evidence that Haygarth's studies were oriented toward medicine at this stage of his education. The rules that governed the awarding of a medical degree had been in force since 1570. The University Statutes stated, "A student of medicine shall learn the medical art by being for six years a constant attendant in the lectures therein, he shall see two dissections, he shall be a respondent twice, and an opponent once (in disputations) before he is made a bachelor." By the beginning of the eighteenth century, however, all that was required of candidates for the degree of Bachelor of Medicine, which Haygarth was to take in 1766, was to keep their names on the college books for five years, reside for nine terms, witness two dissections, and conduct one disputation. By the time he left Cambridge in 1762, John Haygarth would have at least satisfied the residency requirements, and he was at liberty to keep his name on the college list for whatever time he might need to obtain his MB degree.

Edinburgh

It remains unclear why John Haygarth, after his Cambridge years, came to choose medicine as his life's work. Was it his old mathematical teacher, John Dawson, now himself a country practitioner, who suggested a medical career? Did he go to London after leaving Cambridge, where he might have met the more senior Sedbergh alumnus John Fothergill, himself an Edinburgh graduate, who always recommended his alma mater to those intending physicians who so often came to him to seek advice? The previous year Fothergill had advised the young Americans John Morgan of Philadelphia and Arthur Lee of Virginia, future friend of John Haygarth, to attend the medical school in the Scottish capital. Whatever encouragement Haygarth may have received, by the autumn of 1762 he had matriculated at the University of Edinburgh, no doubt attending the ceremony in the library where "the Provost read the formal Latin obligation, asking each of the students to apply himself to his studies, obey the rules of the University and pay respect to its officers, and neither make nor participate in any riot or tumult."[46]

Edinburgh in those days was a crowded city whose habitations clustered around the castle, magnificently sited on Edinburgh's rock, and St. Giles's Cathedral. The New Town had not yet been planned, so that the later efflux of the well-to-do to its elegant Georgian terraces and rows was yet to

[46]Whitfield J. Bell, *John Morgan: Continental Doctor* (Philadelphia: University of Pennsylvania Press, 1965).

come. There were towering tenements that reached as high as twelve stories, courts and wynds upon which the sun never shone, streets crowded with market booths, and people jostling in the thoroughfares in noisy confusion. Sanitation was virtually nonexistent, so being dowsed by household slops thrown into the street from on high was a hazard to which all passersby were exposed. Yet it was a period during which Edinburgh was entering its golden age. It was the city of David Hume and later of Adam Smith, and its university was almost at the highest point of its reputation. Philadelphian Benjamin Rush wrote as a young medical student in 1768, "Tis now at the zenith of its glory. The whole world I believe does not afford a set of greater men than are at present united in the College of Edinburgh."[47]

The medical school that had been founded nearly forty years earlier by Alexander Monro and his fellow students of Herman Boerhaave now attracted students from far and wide. A Danish student wrote of the period when Haygarth was in Edinburgh, "Portugese and Italians, Frenchmen and Englishmen, Irishmen and Dutchmen, Germans and Swiss, Russians and Danes wandered together."[46] They sauntered through Edinburgh's teeming streets as well as its salons and centers of learning. In particular there were numbers of young students from the American Colonies, some like John Morgan and William Shippen seeking to equip themselves for the task of establishing medical education in their own cities and colleges. Arthur Lee, protégé of Benjamin Franklin, paid tribute to the influence of John Fothergill, whose advice he, like other American visitors, had sought after arriving in London in 1760. He wrote that Dr. Fothergill's reputation and knowledge as an Edinburgh graduate who was a successful physician in London had cast such a luster on the status of Edinburgh "that it is now universally resorted to and I believe contains more Physical students than half the Colledges in Europe together with the American Students of whom there is a great number." Lee, devoted as he was to his native land, went further in predicting that "there would one day be a Mead, a Cullen or a Fothergill in America."[48]

As a son of a family of the minor gentry, Haygarth would have found himself among kindred spirits. During those years the majority of the Edinburgh students came from the sons of the "middling ranks, gentry, medical practitioners, military men, ministers and lawyers."[46] They would have lived in reasonable comfort for £10 a quarter, though there were some, enjoying a more fashionable lifestyle, who might have spent as much as £100. Thomas

[47] This account of Edinburgh at the time Haygarth was a student there is taken from ibid.
[48] Bell, "John Morgan."

Ismay was the son of a Yorkshire vicar and therefore similar in background to John Haygarth. He described what £10 a quarter would buy:

> Tea twice a day I chuse; have a Hot Dinner and Supper. The Dinner usually consists of a large *Tirene* of soup, which I like extremely well, a Dish of Boiled Meat and another of Roast. The Mutton and Beef is very good. Veal, I have not seen any yet; puddings only one. Generally to Supper, Fish, Eggs, Beefsteaks or what you leave. Candles what you have occasion for, and a good Fire.[49]

Dinner, taken in the afternoon between three and four, might be got for 6 pence.

Haygarth matriculated for three sessions, 1762–1763, 1763–1764, and 1764–1765. In his first year he enrolled for classes in chemistry and botany, in the following year in anatomy and surgery, botany, chemistry, physiology, and clinical lectures. In his last year he added the practice of medicine to anatomy, surgery, and clinical lectures.[50] His teachers would have included the Monros, father and son, in anatomy, and at the infirmary, where he would visit the sick, his clinical teachers would have been Robert Whytt (1714–1766),[51] William Cullen (1710–1790), and James Gregory (1724–1773).[52] One of the most important parts of the Edinburgh medical course was the clinical instruction at the Edinburgh Royal Infirmary. Clinical teaching already had a long history. In 1539, Givanni da Monte (1498–1561) of the University of Padua brought his students to the Hospital of San Francesco, a practice that was followed in Leiden during the seventeenth century. It was to be a particular feature of Herman Boerhaave's time as professor of medicine in the succeeding century. As Guenter Risse has argued, his bedside teaching at the St. Cecilia Hospital in Leiden set "new standards in medical training." In Edinburgh, the students were advised not to attend the wards until they had received sufficient theoretical instruction. They then had to obtain a ticket that would entitle them to attend clinical lectures and, at set times, to visit patients and copy their case notes.[53] This experience

---

[49] Lisa Rosner, *Medical Education in the Age of Improvement: Edinburgh Students and Apprentices 1760–1826* (Edinburgh: Edinburgh University Press, 1991).

[50] Matriculation records of the University of Edinburgh. Kindly provided by the Library of the University of Edinburgh.

[51] Robert Whytt (1714–1766), *Oxford DNB*, 58:798–799.

[52] James Gregory (1724–1773), *Oxford DNB*, 23:673–675.

[53] Guenter B. Risse, *Hospital Life in Enlightenment Scotland: Care and Teaching at the Royal Infirmary of Edinburgh* (Cambridge: Cambridge University Press, 1986).

undoubtedly gave Haygarth valuable training in the clinical practice of the time. By thc time he left Edinburgh he would not have been overawed by his first encounters with the sick.

Among the talented individuals that the young Haygarth would have encountered at Edinburgh, the most important and influential of his teachers was undoubtedly William Cullen, to whom he was to remain devoted throughout his life. Born in Hamilton, Lanarkshire, in 1710, Cullen graduated with an MD from Glasgow in 1740. He succeeded Dr. Johnstone as professor of medicine at Glasgow University in 1751 but in 1755 was elected professor of chemistry at Edinburgh. His success as a lecturer was immediate. His first course attracted only 17 students, but his second was attended by 59 and soon he had over 140. By 1757 he was also giving clinical lectures at the infirmary. His popularity was enhanced by the fact that he delivered his lectures in English rather than the traditional Latin.[54] He was the great nosologist of his day, presenting his students with a clear and concise categorization of human disease. For the practice of medicine, the student who attended his lectures on clinical medicine would have studied his *First Lines in the Practice of Physic*.[55] The first edition did not appear until 1777, some years after Haygarth was a student, but it is unlikely that Cullen's teaching in earlier years would have differed much from his later publications. Apart from his virtues as a teacher, Cullen was a kindly and warm man who welcomed students to his home.

It would have been from Cullen that Haygarth learned about fevers, the subject that was to consume his interest during his years in active medical practice in Chester. He would have been well aware that for the populace at large and among divines the occurrence of epidemics of disease represented the wrath of god upon unworthy sinners. But although divine retribution was long thought to be the basis for so much human suffering, it was equally understood early in man's experience that disease might be directly infectious, passing by contact from one person to another. This had led to the isolation of the leper as set out in Leviticus. As the years went by, attempts

[54]William Cullen (1710–1790), *Oxford DNB;* 5:277–284. See also A. Doig, J.P.S. Ferguson, I. A. Milne, and R. Passmore, *William Cullen and the Eighteenth Century Medical World* (Edinburgh: Edinburgh University Press, 1993). For Cullen on fever, see W. F. Bynum, "Cullen and the Study of Fevers in Britain," in *Theories of Fever from Antiquity to the Enlightenment*, ed. W. F. Bynum and V. Nutton *Medical History,* supplement no. 1 (London: Wellcome Institute for the History of Medicine, 1981).

[55]William Cullen, *First Lines in the Practice of Physic: For the Students of the University of Edinburgh* (Edinburgh: William Creed and J. Morris, 1777).

were made to control other diseases by isolation. The first quarantine regulations came into force in the Venetian port of Ragusa (now Dubrovnik) in the last years of the fourteenth century after the disaster of the Black Death, and the lazarettos of the Mediterranean ports were specifically intended to prevent the spread of plague.

At the same time, there were many who considered that epidemic fevers were due to something in the atmosphere that all men breathe.[56] The Hippocratic writers, opposing a religious or miraculous explanation of disease with an attempt at something more natural, considered, "Whenever the air has been tainted with such pollution [*miasmasin*] as are hostile to the human race men fall sick."[56] The pollution of the air, it came to be thought, was due to putrefaction of animal and plant substances in the earth, the emanations from the refuse of slaughterhouses, or the unpleasant smell that hangs over marshes. Whatever produced the atmospheric miasmata, it was from something noisome in the air that infection might come. As an old version of a mediaeval poem put it,

> Though all savours do not breed infection
> Yet true infection cometh most by smelling.[56]

The London physician Thomas Sydenham (1624–1689), self-proclaimed protagonist of the Hippocratic tradition, followed the Greek view. Infection, he thought, was due to agents consisting "almost entirely of decayed or diseased organic substances, and of animal emanations or secretions . . . found to exist most abundantly in marshy and alluvial soils, in slaughterhouses, common sewers, dissecting rooms, graveyards, and in those places where a large number of living persons are gathered together, particularly if the effluvia of their secretions taint the atmosphere."[56] Sydenham's views had an almost Galenical influence on medical thinking during his own time and during the next century. Richard Mead, in his *Discourse Concerning Pestilential Contagion*, published in 1720, considered that in the case of plague, "When the constitution of the Air happens to favour Infection, it rages with great violence."[57] Even at the end of the eighteenth century, Patrick Russell, later to be one of Haygarth's nominators for

[56] Owsei Temkin, "An Historical Analysis of the Concept of Infection," in *The Double Face of Janus and Other Essays in the History of Medicine,* ed. Temkin (Baltimore and London: Johns Hopkins University Press, 1977).

[57] Richard Mead, *A Short Discourse Concerning Pestilential Contagion and the Methods to be Used to Prevent it* (London: S. Buckley, 1720).

the fellowship of the Royal Society, wrote that plague was contracted from "substances having imbibed the pestiferous miasmata."[58]

The terms "miasma" and "contagion" have changed through the centuries. As Margaret Pelling has put it, "Ideas of contagion are inseparable from notions of individual morality, social responsibility and collective action." The concept of miasma is, like contagion, "an idea of great antiquity and of shifting allusion over time, its original Greek meaning related to pollution or polluting agent."[59]

It is little wonder that practitioners of medicine of Haygarth's time would be confused by the theories of fever that abounded. Edinburgh students of that era, however, were fortunate in their teacher. William Cullen taught them that, following his own nosology, the class Pyrexiae included five orders: fevers, inflammations, eruptions, haemorrhages, and fluxes. As to the causes of such afflictions, Cullen followed traditional thought, recognizing that "some matter floating in the atmosphere and applied to the bodies of man, ought to be considered as the . . . cause of fever. These matters, present in the atmosphere, may be considered either MIASMA or CONTAGIONS." Miasma, he told his pupils, "arises from marsh or moist ground, acted upon by heat" and is in general a cause of intermittent fever. Contagion was the cause of jail and hospital fever. In such cases the virulent state of human effluvia was responsible. Miasmata might, however, be due not only to the effluvia of marshes but to human effluvia. In respect of specific diseases, Cullen was a model of clarity. He taught that plague always arose as a result of contagion; for this reason prevention by quarantine and by other regulations of the civic authority were required. Smallpox he considered "a contagion of a specific nature." He described the technique of inoculation but said nothing on isolation. Other diseases, such as chickenpox, measles, and scarlet fever, as well as the malignant sore throat (diphtheria), were all due to a specific contagion, as was the "Chin-cough" (whooping cough).[60] By the time Haygarth reached Chester after his Edinburgh training, he must have had a fair understanding of contemporary ideas on fever.

John Haygarth made many friends while a medical student in Edinburgh. Anthony Fothergill, also a Sedbergh School alumnus, had graduated MD in 1763, at the end of Haygarth's first year. His immediate contemporaries

[58] Patrick Russell, *A Treatise of the Plague* (London: GGJ and J. Robinson, 1721).

[59] Margaret Pelling, "Contagion/Germ Theory/Specificity," in *Companion Encyclopedia of the History of Medicine,* ed. W. F. Bynum and Roy Porter (London and New York: Routledge, 1993), 309–334. See also: Caroline Hannaway. Environment and Miasmata. Ibid, pp 292–308.

[60] Cullen, *First Lines.*

included Thomas Percival from Warrington, William Withering, later of Birmingham, and William Falconer, son of the recorder of Chester. Nathaniel Hulme, the first physician to the Aldersgate Dispensary, founded by Lettsom in 1770, was in Haygarth's year. But many of his closest friends seem to have been Americans. Five of his immediate contemporaries were from the American Colonies—Samuel Bard of Philadelphia, Corbin Griffin of Virginia, and Thomas Ruston, James Tapscott, and Samuel Martin.[61] So close were his American friendships that when he was elected a member of the Royal Medical Society, the oldest and most respected of Edinburgh's student societies, his entry was listed among "American members."[62]

His closest friend, however, was Arthur Lee, one of the aristocratic Lees of Virginia, who had been subjected to Samuel Johnson's conservative views on medical education in London in 1760. It was at that time that he had met and been so favorably impressed by John Fothergill, friend and physician to Benjamin Franklin, who had been in London since 1757. It is not surprising that Fothergill, who had close links with Philadelphia Quakers, was also a strong supporter of the American cause and of individual Americans in the years that led to independence. American visitors, particularly the young, had a standing invitation to breakfast with him.

Lee was a botanist of great ability, winning the university's botany prize for his *Hortus siccus* in 1763.[63] In Edinburgh he was a particular friend of Lord Cardross, later the Earl of Buchan, who like Fothergill was highly sympathetic to Americans and their spirit of independence. The American students in Edinburgh had a reputation for hard work. Many of them had a deep interest in the future of their chosen profession in their native colonies. John Morgan went on to found the first medical school in America, in Philadelphia, in 1765. Lee himself was particularly concerned with the standards of medical practice in his native Virginia. The Americans therefore had an interest in ensuring that the Edinburgh degree that many of them took would be recognized as of the highest standing, so when in 1764 two individuals who had not fulfilled the university's requirements were awarded degrees, Lee courageously persuaded twenty-nine of his fellow students, mostly Americans, to sign a memorial to the professors protesting the faculty's actions. The professors responded by refusing the degree to one student but

[61] *List of Graduates in Medicine in the University of Edinburgh* (Edinburgh: Neill & Company, 1867).

[62] Information provided by Patricia E. Strong, permanent secretary, Royal Medical Society, Edinburgh.

[63] Bell, *Arthur Lee.*

agreeing to the other, a compromise that satisfied only some of the rebels. Naturally there was great concern on both sides. Lee himself felt impelled to write a personal letter to William Cullen. "My conduct in public," he wrote, "tho' rash, I am satisfied has been sincere & honourable. But should it induce Dr Cullen to think, that I have never felt or have ungratefully forgot the duties I owe to his uncommon goodness; it will add the highest affliction, to the concern which I already feel."[64] Needless to say, it was his own degree that most concerned Lee, but to his relief he was duly awarded his MD in the summer of 1764, his thesis entitled *De Cortico Peruviano*. He stayed on in Edinburgh for another year after his graduation. It was not, however, the end of the argument over the Edinburgh degree. In 1766, Samuel Leeds, who was illiterate in Latin, was awarded his MD for a thesis entitled *De Asthmate Spasmodico*, even though it was later shown that his thesis had not been his own. In London, John Fothergill, defending the interests of those like himself with an Edinburgh degree, became deeply involved in litigation over the question of how Leeds had obtained his doctorate.[65]

Haygarth, with his American sympathies, no doubt supported his fellow students, but at the end of his three years in Edinburgh he did not take a degree, presumably because he was intending to return to Cambridge to graduate. It was probably Arthur Lee who now suggested to him that they should undertake a continental tour. Lee had written from Edinburgh to his brother in Virginia the previous summer, "It is my plan at present to remain here this winter, to set out early in the spring for Leyden, where I shall not make a very long stay, but proceed to Paris & whatever German Universities may be worth visiting."[66] It must have been spring, as Lee had hoped, when they set off, taking with them an older fellow student, John Berkenhout, the son of a prosperous Dutch merchant, who was from Leeds in Yorkshire. Berkenhout was well known to Lee, for he had signed the letter to the professors objecting to the irregularities in awarding degrees. Berkenhout's linguistic skills must have proved valuable to the trio. All three matriculated at Leiden University on May 13, 1765, but only Berkenhout, who like Haygarth had not graduated in Edinburgh, took a Leiden degree. Normally any English student would have signed the matriculation roll and added "Anglicus." Not Haygarth, who emphasized his origins in an obscure valley of the Yorkshire

[64] Autograph letter, Arthur Lee to William Cullen, 18 April 1764, Cullen–Thomson papers, Glasgow University Library.

[65] Fox. *Dr John Fothergill and His Friends.*

[66] Autograph letter, Arthur Lee to R. H. Lee, Edinburgh, Sept 1, 1764, Lee Papers, University of Virginia.

dales by proudly writing "Garsdala-Anglicus."[67] It seems to have been a highly successful trip. For John Haygarth, it was a period of great pleasure. Forty years later, in a letter to colleagues in Philadelphia, he remembered his "intimate friend" Arthur Lee, with whom he had spent "many agreeable hours at Edinburgh, London, Leiden and Paris."[68]

Lee stayed on in London after their return and did not set out for Virginia until the following year. John Haygarth apparently also stayed in London, attending one of the hospitals and extending his Edinburgh clinical experience. It seems highly likely that he would have visited John Fothergill with Lee during this time. He may well also have paid a visit to his native Garsdale, where his property interests had grown. In 1762, he had been left much of the remainder of his grandfather's estate upon the death of his uncle Richard, elder brother of his father. His legacy included the old family home at Swarthgill.

Whatever he did during 1766, he must at some time have returned to Cambridge, where he received his Bachelor of Medicine degree (Cantab). He never took a Cambridge MD and only became an MD thirty years later when he was honored by another college, this time in Cambridge, Massachusetts, which had duly become Harvard University.

[67] *Album Studiosorum Academiae Lugdano Batavae MDLXXV–MDCCCLXXV* (Hagae Comitum: Apud Martinum Nijhoff, 1875), 1086.

[68] Autograph letter, John Haygarth to the Gentlemen of the College, Bath, 6 October 1806, courtesy of the College of Physicians of Philadelphia.

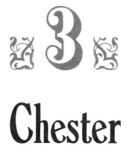

Chester

Physician to the Chester Infirmary

*I*n 1767 John Haygarth moved to Chester, where he was to spend the next thirty-one years as a provincial physician, years that were to establish his reputation. Here he undertook the work that led to his election as a fellow of the Royal Society. The city that became his home and where he brought up his family had its origins in Roman times.[69] In the first century AD the Romans founded Deva, one of their main fortresses in Britain, on the site of the present city of Chester in a loop of the River Dee. As a port it was to be a base for the Roman fleet in the north of England. For 200 years the Twentieth Valeria Victrix Legion served at Deva. In Anglo-Saxon times Chester became a prosperous and rich community with its thriving port on the River Dee. After the Norman Conquest it became an important center, under the Earl of Chester, for mounting expeditions against the rebellious Welsh. It effectively became a city-state in the fifteenth century, but by the end of the Civil War, when it suffered from its support of the Royalist cause, the city's prosperity had begun to decline. Thereafter the port gradually silted up, leaving Liverpool to become the major port in the northwest of England, providing imported cotton in particular for the emerging industries of Manchester. By the time John Haygarth arrived in Chester in 1767, the city was still relatively prosperous. There was, however, to be none of the major development of industry or population growth that were so much a feature of nearby Manchester or Liverpool, where industrialization was associated with dramatic increases in population during the second half of the eighteenth century. Chester had always had strong royal connections—after all, the Prince of Wales was, as he still is, traditionally Earl of Chester—and in

[69] *Chester Official Guide* (Chester: Chester City Council, 1985).

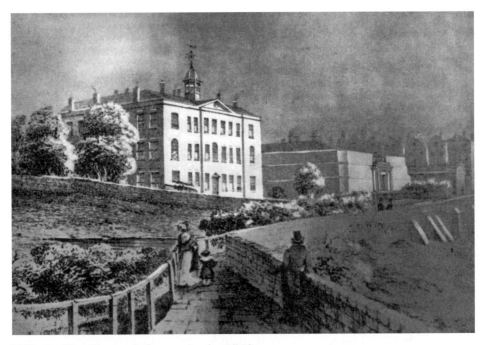

FIG. 3. The Chester Infirmary in the 1760s.
(Courtesy of the Countess of Chester Hospital NHS Trust.)

national politics it was supportive of traditional Tory values. The city, which preserved its ancient walls, was largely in the hands of the Grosvenor family, who controlled the city's two Tory seats in the House of Commons.[70]

It may well have been John Haygarth's friendship with his fellow Edinburgh student William Falconer that led him to settle in Chester. William Falconer's father, also William, was the recorder of Chester and therefore part of the Grosvenor oligarchy that controlled the affairs of the town. Sir Richard Grosvenor, later first Earl Grosvenor, was the first chairman of the charity that founded the Chester Infirmary in 1755. William Falconer senior was also one of the founders of the charity and he held the important position of treasurer. His son Thomas, elder brother of Dr. William, became a governor of the charity in 1765 and was also chairman of weekly board meetings at the time of John Haygarth's election as a physician in 1767. Haygarth, a Cambridge graduate and practicing Anglican, may well have appealed to the traditional elements among those responsible for infirmary

[70] Lobo, "John Haygarth."

appointments. As in other provincial cities throughout the land, however, Edinburgh was an important training ground for its physicians. It is significant that Haygarth's friend William Falconer, MD of Edinburgh in 1766, became a physician to the infirmary at the same time as Haygarth. Other Edinburgh graduates, such as William Currie, cousin of Haygarth's Liverpool friend James Currie, were practicing in Chester at the time.[71] William Falconer remained a close friend of John Haygarth throughout his life, even though he resigned his position in 1769 to move to Bath the following year, apparently at the suggestion of John Fothergill.

At its foundation in 1755, the infirmary was housed in the upper part of the Blue-Coat School, outside the Northgate.[72] Its first patient was one William Thompson of St. Mary's Parish, who was admitted with a wounded hand on November 11, 1755. The original medical staff included three physicians and three surgeons. The board of governors, which also included the medical staff, was responsible for the admission and discharge of patients. As with other foundations throughout the land, to be admitted required a letter from a subscriber or a person of good repute, such as a clergyman. For 2 guineas a year a subscriber could recommend one inpatient and two outpatients. The premises at the Blue-Coat School soon became hopelessly overcrowded, and in 1761 (the date can still be seen inscribed above the main door) a new purpose-built building was erected on open ground within the city walls. When Haygarth and Falconer were appointed to the staff, they joined the two physicians who had been there since the foundation of the infirmary, neither of whom has emerged from obscurity. One was Edward Weaver, whose MD cannot now be traced, and the other was Alexander Denton, MD of Rheims.[73] With the arrival of the two young men from Edinburgh, both of whom were to be elected fellows of the Royal Society, the standing of physicians in Chester was to increase greatly.

Haygarth first lived in Watergate Street. In January 1776, however, he bound himself to the Lord Bishop of Chester in the sum of 100 pounds in order to obtain a license to marry Sarah Vere Widdens. His future wife was the daughter of William Widdens of Chistleton, Cheshire, Gentleman.[74] After

[71]Thornton, *James Currie, The Entire Stranger and Robert Burns* (Edinburgh and London: Oliver and Boyd, 1963).

[72]E. M. Mumford, *Chester Royal Infirmary 1756–1956* (Chester: Chester and District Hospital Management Committee, 1956).

[73]P. J. Wallis and R. V. Wallis, *Eighteenth Century Medics (Subscriptions, Licences, Apprenticeships)* (Newcastle upon Tyne: Project for Historical Biobibliography, 1988).

[74]Information from Cheshire Record Office.

their marriage, John and Sarah Haygarth moved to Foregate Street, where they built a substantial house, no longer preserved, with a large garden that extended as far as the Chester Canal. Haygarth seems to have made extensions to the property in 1784, when he bought part of an adjacent "jousting croft." The instructions that he gave to Charles Potts, his lawyer, on that occasion illustrate the blunt and forthright way in which he expressed himself, and not only on medical matters:

> I wish you to offer Mr Turner the very extravagant sum of 500 £ for that portion of the justing croft which lies on the east side of the line that would be made by continuing the west wall of my garden, in a straight direction, to the Canal. This price is the highest I shall ever offer and indeed much higher than was ever before thought of by your obliged and faithful servant

> John Haygarth[75]

Haygarth and his wife had six children. As was common in those days, several did not survive infancy or childhood. Their first child, Elizabeth, was born in 1777 but died in infancy. Mary Widdens Haygarth, however, born at the end of that year, was to live on until her 70s, dying during the reign of Queen Victoria. Ann was born in 1779 and Sarah Vere Widdens three years later. Both died in childhood, one of them perhaps in 1787, when Haygarth's old student friend, Thomas Percival, wrote from Manchester. "I need not express to my dear Friend my cordial sympathy with him on this melancholy occasion. . . . Indulge your tears," he wrote, "Jesus wept for Lazarus."[76] There were then two sons, who lived to brighten their father's declining years. William was born on January 18, 1784, and his brother John in November 1786. As befitted the family of a committed Anglican, the children were all baptized in the Holy Trinity Church in Chester.[77] Throughout his years in Chester, John Haygarth kept in close touch with his family in his native Garsdale. His properties there had to be managed, of course, a task undertaken for some years by his half-brother Leonard. His immaculate accounts from 1788 to 1802 have been preserved and show both the rents John Haygarth received from his properties and the expenses

---

[75] Autograph letter, John Haygarth to Charles Potts, Cheshire Record Office.

[76] Edward Percival, *Memoirs of the Life and Writings of Thomas Percival: To which is added a selection of his Literary Correspondence* (Bath: R. Crutwell, 1807), cxx.

[77] Parish Records of the Church of the Holy and Undivided Trinity of the City of Chester.

incurred by Leonard in running them.[78] By the end of that period Haygarth owned the family home at Swarthgill, as well as farms nearby at Birkrigg, Fawcetts, and Castley. He also owned Garsdale Hall, later an inn. His net rental income was more than £170 a year, but there were constant bills for walling and slating, repairs to stable doors, pointing of chimneys, and the like. The Chester family clearly relied on Garsdale for provisions, as repeated orders for hams (at 6 1/2 pence a pound in 1788), hung beef, and strong cheeses appear in the accounts. In March 1793, Haygarth was charged the remarkable sum of £35 for a "young horse including Man's Exps to Chester." Bills made out to Mr. Wakefield in London no doubt represent the banking of Haygarth's profits, paid through the bank of the Quaker Wakefields of Kendal, a mere ten miles from Sedbergh.

He also kept in close touch with his old mathematical teacher and Garsdale friend, John Dawson, who was frequently consulted by Haygarth on mathematical questions relating to his studies of smallpox and other fevers. John Haygarth seems to have had a gift for friendship and he made many other friends during his years in Chester. His close relationship with William Falconer and the Falconer family continued long after William resigned from the Chester Infirmary in 1769 to settle in Bath. In June 1772, Haygarth wrote to his old teacher, William Cullen, to introduce Thomas Falconer, elder brother of the physician.[79] Thomas Falconer had been called to the bar at Lincoln's Inn in 1760 but ill-health precluded him from practice. He lived a life of studious retirement in Chester, where he became known for his interest in antiquities and for his patronage of literature. Dr. Johnson's Lichfield friend, the poetess Anna Seward, referred to him as the "Maecenas of Chester." Haygarth's letter to Cullen read as follows:

> As I have always observed that men of superior abilities entertain a particular regard and esteem for each other, I think myself extremely fortunate in having an opportunity of introducing to you Mr Falconer, brother to the Doctor, your late pupil. You will soon find that Mr Falconer has acquired an uncommon degree of knowledge in every branch of both ancient and modern learning, and in natural history. He is very desirous of becoming personally acquainted with the men of genius of our sister kingdom, who have become so justly celebrated

[78] Accounts kept by Leonard Haygarth, 1788–1802, Badgerdub Papers, in the possession of Denise Colton, Badgerdub Cottage, Garsdale. Leonard Haygarth died in 1802. There is a tablet to his memory in Garsdale Church.

[79] Thomas Falconer (1738–1792), *Oxford DNB;* 18:973.

for their excellent publications in every part of polite literature; and, on this account, I think myself most fortunate in introducing him to one who is so intimately known, and so highly respected by them all.

Your old pupil thinks himself extremely happy in having an opportunity of returning his most grateful acknowledgements for the most useful instructions he has received from Dr Cullen as his professor, and for the innumerable kind offices he has experienced from him as a friend. Old physicians generally complain that practice contradicts the theories they had been taught to trust with implicit faith in their medical schools. The reverse seems likely to be my case. In the study of physic, I was very sceptical in admitting theories, and can now, with truth, observe that most of the general doctrines I then adopted, particularly those of Dr Cullen, have been rather confirmed than confuted by practice. The cause of this difference seems very obvious. I continue, with increasing respect and esteem, your most grateful pupil

John Haygarth[80]

Apart from illustrating the high regard Haygarth held for William Cullen, the letter shows how as a provincial physician Haygarth was concerned in Chester not only with medicine. He also maintained his friendship with those local intellectuals who were involved in the life of his adopted city and who were to support him in his efforts to help his fellow citizens.

Many of Haygarth's medical friends were dissenters, to the extent that Lobo has claimed that Haygarth, although an Anglican, was part of a network of dissenters in the northwest of England at that time. In 1770, William Currie, from a Dumfries family, newly graduated from Edinburgh, moved to Chester to practice. His cousin, James Currie, came to Liverpool some years later and there developed his interest in the treatment of fever with cold water douches and the use of the clinical thermometer. Currie became a Unitarian and was a firm supporter of radical causes. Other Liverpool physicians and Edinburgh graduates who became Haygarth's friends included Matthew Dobson, James Rutter, and James Bostock.[81]

The Unitarian Manchester physician Thomas Percival,[82] Haygarth's exact contemporary, was originally an Anglican but then became a pupil at the famous Warrington Academy, a haven for dissenters where the Unitarian

[80] John Thomson, *An Account of the Life, Lectures and Writings of William Cullen* (Edinburgh and London: William Blackwood and Sons, 1859), 638.

[81] R. D. Thornton, *James Currie, The Entire Stranger and Robert Burns* (Edinburgh and London: Oliver and Boyd, 1963).

[82] Thomas Percival MD (1740–1804), *Oxford DNB;* 43:675–676.

Joseph Priestley taught. A classmate of Haygarth at Edinburgh, Percival had spent a year in London while still a student and had made the acquaintance of many scientific men, among them Lord Willoughby, vice president of the Royal Society. Through his influence Percival was elected a fellow of the society, apparently the youngest man at that time on whom that honor had been conferred. Percival graduated MD at Leiden in 1765. He wrote to William Cullen in November 1770 telling him that his old Edinburgh students, Bostock, Dobson, Haygarth, and himself, "have agreed to meet, for our mutual improvement, every three months at Warrington, which lies in the centre between Liverpool, Chester and Manchester. Glad shall I be to receive any medical intelligence from you that I may communicate to our Society."[83] Percival, later to be known for his *Medical Ethics*,[84] founded the Manchester Literary and Philosophical Society in 1781, conducting meetings in a Unitarian Chapel. Haygarth made two contributions to the society, one in collaboration with Thomas Henry, the Unitarian chemist, titled, "On the preservation of Sea Water from putrefaction by means of quicklime; with an account of a newly invented machine for impregnating water and other fluids with fixed Air, &c."[85] Haygarth, like his old teacher John Dawson, was to become an honorary member of the Manchester society. Others who enjoyed Haygarth's friendship included the Edinburgh trained physician and notorious Unitarian John Aikin, whose father had been one of the founders of the Warrington Academy.

Thomas Percival was, however, the closest of Haygarth's medical friends. They corresponded on many subjects other than medicine: financial support for Dr. Priestley, John Howard's proposal to bring forward a bill to support the use of liquors in prisons, and queries from Percival as to what exertions were being made at Chester "to suppress the Slave Trade." Percival also chided him for his "neglect of your duty as an honorary member of the Institute," the Manchester Literary and Philosophical Society. "I wish you would send us some communication," he wrote. There was also a plea for Haygarth to send his "stricture on my taxation essay," a piece that to this day is a long and complicated document. They were concerned with Voltaire and his friends, whose infidelity arose "from the zeal to emancipate

[83]Thomson. *William Cullen,* 635.

[84]Thomas Percival, *Medical Ethics:or a code of Institutes and Precepts adapted to the Professional Conduct of Physicians and Surgeons* (Manchester: J. Russell; London: J. Johnson, 1803).

[85]John Haygarth, "On the preservation of Sea Water from putrefaction by means of quicklime; with an account of a newly invented machine for impregnating water and other fluids with fixed Air, &c," *Memoirs of the Manchester Literary and Philosophical Society* 1 (1785): 51–54.

themselves from all the nurse and all the priest had taught." After Percival's death, when his son Edward published a memoir of his life together with his writings and selections from his correspondence, he dedicated the work to John Haygarth. He wrote, "Your friendship he valued among the earliest, the most durable, and the most affectionate which his life afforded."[86]

It may well have been with Arthur Lee in London in 1766 that Haygarth first met the famous Quaker physician, John Fothergill. He was, however, to become more closely acquainted with him during his early years in Chester. In 1765, Dr. Fothergill and his sister Ann, who acted as his housekeeper, sought a retreat in the country where they could escape from their increasingly frenetic life in London. They chose Lea Hall, a square-built house of the Queen Anne period, near Middlewich in Cheshire, 150 miles from London and conveniently situated near Warrington, where their preacher brother, Samuel, lived.[87] Here they spent two months every summer, ensured for a little while of relief from the fatigue of London life and able, as the doctor put it, "to recover the power of recollection."[88] Here Haygarth would visit, on at least one occasion taking his Manchester friend, Thomas Percival, with him. Whether these visits were always appreciated by the Fothergills is uncertain. In 1771, the doctor wrote to his brother in Warrington that Drs. Haygarth and Percival "spent yesterday and part of the night with us and exhausted me not a little."[89]

There were, however, other advantages of Haygarth's visits to Lea Hall. In the summer of 1769, he met Fothergill's protégé, John Coakley Lettsom, who was to remain a firm friend and supporter. In 1778 he also met the doctor's American cousin, Benjamin Waterhouse, then a medical student in Edinburgh. Waterhouse, later a close correspondent of Haygarth, became the first professor of medicine at the college that had become Harvard

---

[86] Percival, *Memoirs.*

[87] Samuel Fothergill (1715–1772) was a much valued Quaker preacher who like his father traveled in the ministry to the American Colonies. He settled in the business of a tea dealer and American merchant in Warrington. Fox, *Dr John Fothergill and His Friends*, 239–250.

[88] Booth, "Ann Fothergill."

[89] Corner and Booth, *Chain of Friendship.*

FIG. 4. **a.** William Heberden;
   b. John Fothergill;
   c. Benjamin Waterhouse;
   d. William Withering *(All courtesy of the Wellcome Library, London.)*

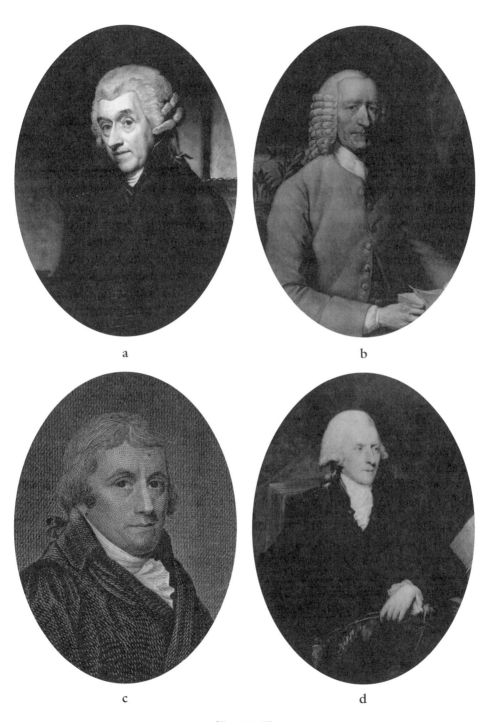

a

b

c

d

University. It was he who in 1795 obtained the honorary degree of MD for his old friend from Chester.[90]

It may well have been other than purely medical questions that occupied Dr. Fothergill when Haygarth came to visit. In the summer of 1772, Haygarth must have been reminded of his efforts with Arthur Lee when they were students in Edinburgh to maintain the standard of the Edinburgh degree. During that year Fothergill was involved in a series of lawsuits that concerned the fraudulent degree obtained in Edinburgh by a fellow Quaker, Samuel Leeds, then seeking to establish himself in practice in London. Fothergill wrote that summer from Lea Hall to William Cullen, sending his brother Alexander, who had some legal training, to seek help and obtain affidavits that would expose Leeds as an imposter.[91]

It was also in 1772 that John Haygarth persuaded Fothergill to join the many citizens of Chester who petitioned the monarch for an act to make a "Navigable Cut or Canal from the River Dee, within the liberties of the City of Chester, to run near Middlewich and Nantwich, in the County of Chester."[92] Alexander Denton, Haygarth's colleague at the Chester Infirmary, was another supporter. It was to be an unsuccessful venture until incorporated with the Ellesmere Canal in 1805.[93]

John Haygarth's clinical practice in Chester included the patients he cared for in the course of his duties as a physician to the infirmary. The records of the infirmary have been preserved and include diagnoses of the many patients who sought help. Their ailments were many and varied, including asthma, consumption, jaundice, dropsy, scrofula, scurvy, worms, and apparently leprosy (a term then used not for the biblical condition but for a variety of scaly disorders of the skin), as well as hysterics in a number of women. In addition, Haygarth kept careful records of the many patients he saw during his practice outside the hospital. He constantly recorded, he wrote later, "in the patient's chamber, a full and accurate account of every important symptom, the remedies which

[90] Information provided by Richard J. Wolfe, Francis A. Countway Library of Medicine, Harvard Medical Library.

[91] Corner and Booth, *Chain of Friendship*.

[92] Chester Canal Act (1772), 12 Geo III. Haygarth attended the subscribers meeting in 1770 and subscribed £200 for himself. The first meetings were chaired by his colleague at the Chester Infirmary, Dr. Denton. Information provided by Professor T. J. Peters, a biochemist from Kings College Hospital Medical School and enthusiastic owner of a canal boat in Cheshire, who interests himself in the history of canals.

[93] Charles Hadfield, *British Canals: An Illustrated History*, 6th ed. (Newton Abbot, London, North Pomfret: David & Charles, 1979), 102–103.

were employed, and when an opportunity offered, the effects which they produced." He noted and classed the cases of 10,549 patients, as well as those of "a large number of persons in the lower ranks of life."[94] It is a matter of regret that his records have not been preserved.

As the years went by, Haygarth seems to have achieved a notable reputation. We are given a tantalizing glimpse of him as a physician in the 1790s, by which time he had become firmly established in Chester. Mrs. Thrale, Dr. Johnson's frequent hostess, writing at Streatham on October 20, 1792, recorded that her niece Cecilia Thrale had "catched a dreadful cold in the rain" when they were in Wales and her cough was "Furious." "We sent for Haygarth from Chester," she went on, "he is a famous physician—and he bled her copiously." Three years later, that same Cecilia, having made a runaway marriage with John Mostyn, was "frightened into fits on her wedding night. . . . Her husband kindly and considerately got Dr Haygarth to prescribe for her at Chester."[95] These visits were no doubt carefully recorded by Haygarth among the copious notes he took great trouble in making.

He seems to have visited patients at a distance from Chester, particularly in North Wales. On one occasion he had a remarkable experience. In February 1780, he was returning to Chester from a visit to St. Asaph and on ascending at Rhealt, the mountain which forms the eastern boundary of the Vale of Clwyd, he observed a rare and curious phenomenon:

> In the road above me I was struck with the peculiar appearance of a very white shining cloud, that lay remarkably close to the ground. I walked up to the cloud, and my shadow was projected into it; when, a very unexpected and beautiful scene was presented to my view. The head of my shadow was surrounded, at some distance, by a circle of various colours, whose centre appeared to be near the situation of the eye, and the whole circumference extended to the shoulders. The circle was complete, except what the shadow of my body intercepted. It exhibited the most vivid colours, red being outermost: as far as can be recollected, all the colours appeared in the same order and proportion that the rain-bow presents to our view. It resembled, very exactly, what in pictures is termed a *glory*, around the head of our Saviour, and of saints: not indeed that luminous radiance, which is painted close to the head, but an arch of concentric colours, which is placed separate and

[94] John Haygarth, *A Clinical History of Disease. I: A Clinical History of Acute Rhaeumatism: II. A Clinical History of the Nodosity if the Joints* (Bath: R. Crutwell, 1805).

[95] Katherine C. Balderstone, *The Diary of Mrs. Hester Thrale* (Oxford: Clarendon Press, 1942).

distinct from it. As I walked forward, this *glory* approached or retired, just as the inequality of the ground shortened or lengthened my shadow. The cloud being sometimes in the small valley below me, sometimes on the same level, or on higher ground, the variation of the shadow, and *glory* became extremely striking and singular.[96]

Haygarth went on to describe the right and left arches of a white shining bow, not joined to a semicircle. Later that same evening he was passing through a similar cloud when he noticed that icicles had formed on his hair, "which by the motion of riding, produced a sound, like the ringing of distant bells." While Haygarth supposed that the "glory," or halo around his head, was caused by light shining on tiny frozen particles in a cloud, what he was seeing is now known as the Brocken bow or Brocken specter. It is so named because at the highest point of the Harz Mountains in Germany, called Brocken, shadows cast from the peak become magnified when the sun is low and seemingly gigantic silhouettes are cast upon the upper surfaces of low-lying clouds or fog below the mountain. Haygarth's careful observations were read by Percival in a paper to the Manchester Literary and Philosophical Society on March 13, 1789, and were accompanied by a drawing made by his Chester friend, Thomas Falconer. Percival wrote later from Manchester to let him know that "your paper concerning the Glory was unanimously balloted for inclusion in the third volume of the Memoirs of the Society."[97] Samuel Taylor Coleridge witnessed the same phenomenon during a walking tour of the Harz Mountains in 1799. He described the experience in his poem "Constancy to an ideal object," in which the woodman

> Sees full before him, gliding without tread,
> An image with a glory round its head.[98]

While Haygarth's more religious friends might well have interpreted what he saw as a sign of divine approval, it was characteristic that, devout Anglican though he was, no such thought ever entered his head.

[96] John Haygarth, "Description of a Glory," *Memoirs of the Manchester Literary and Philosophical Society* 3 (1790): 463–466.

[97] Percival, *Memoirs*, cxl.

[98] *The Poetical Works of S. T. Coleridge. Reprinted from the early editions with Memoir, Notes etc.* (London and New York: Frederick Warne and Co., n.d.), 234. There is a reference to Haygarth's paper in a footnote to this work.

The Population and Diseases of Chester

One of the earliest of Haygarth's activities as a physician in Chester was to undertake a study of the population and diseases of his chosen city. There were others throughout the land at that time who were interested in establishing registers of births, marriages, deaths, and causes of death, but one of the first to attempt to obtain legislation to set up such registers was John Fothergill, and it may well have been he, during Haygarth's summer visits to his country home at Lea Hall, who encouraged Haygarth. It is significant that Thomas Percival, another summer visitor to Lea Hall, was at the same time engaging in similar studies in Manchester.

As early as 1754, Fothergill had taken steps to bring the need for a proper registration of births, burials, and causes of death before the authorities.[99] The weekly Bills of Mortality in London had been in existence since the time of Queen Elizabeth, yet they were totally inaccurate. Searchers, mostly poor ignorant women, viewed the bodies of the dead and assigned a cause of death to them. There were three main categories: consumptions, convulsions, and fevers. Any emaciated body was debited to consumption, so that London earned an undeservedly bad name as an unhealthy city. The system was under the control of the parish clerks in London, and to them Fothergill proposed that there should be exact registers of births, deaths and marriages, not only in the London parishes within the city of London, but also throughout the land. In order better to record the causes of death, Fothergill brought together a group of eminent physicians to make a comprehensive and understandable list of causes of death that could be used by those responsible for reporting deaths. The Company of Parish Clerks was sufficiently impressed by Fothergill's proposal to apply to Parliament for powers to carry it into effect. Thomas Potter MP undertook the task of proposing the measures to the House of Commons, and a bill was printed that seemed likely to have a fair wind. Unfortunately, Potter insisted that there be a census of the people of both sexes and ages before the other provisions came into effect, something that was not to take place until 1801, when the first national census was taken. The opposition in Parliament was outraged and assailed this new clause with great clamor. As Fothergill put it, "Nothing but the Sin of David was heard of."[100] Unfortunately for Fothergill, the bill was rejected by a large majority.

---

[99] Fox, *Dr. Fothergill and His Friends*, 227–229.

[100] After King David carried out a census of the people of Israel, his "heart smote him. . . . And David said unto the Lord I have sinned greatly in what I have done" 2 Samuel 24:10. The reason why the census was sinful is obscure.

Yet Fothergill clearly continued to press the cause of national registers. In 1768, he gave a paper to his fellow members of the Society of Physicians, which he had founded, recounting in detail the events of 1754 and apologizing to them that although the matter under consideration was not specifically about something medical, it was of significance to all physicians. In 1771, the year he recorded that Haygarth and Percival had visited him at Lea Hall "and exhausted me not a little," he wrote to his Quaker correspondent in Philadelphia, James Pemberton,

> I wish your Province would establish a general Register of births, burials and marriages—to have an officer, some person who can write and read in every township, to register these circumstances within a few days after the fact, and to transmit the account to Philadelphia annually. Much useful information would accrue from it. If you once think of it seriously, I will send a copy of a bill brought into Parliament some years ago, and the reason for its miscarriage.[101]

John Haygarth made a detailed study of the Bills of Mortality in Chester for 1772, 1773, and 1774. He, like Fothergill, was clearly concerned that the causes of death should be accurate and understandable to all and sundry. The board of the Chester Infirmary, upon which his friend Thomas Falconer sat, was undoubtedly interested in the work, for the assembly book records that Dr. Haygarth was paid 10 guineas for his survey of the "inhabitants, annual births and deaths relating to the healthiness of the situation."[102] The influence of his Edinburgh mentor, William Cullen, was evident, as Haygarth pointed out that

> In the Table of diseases...the technical are added to the vulgar names, and the arrangement of a justly celebrated professor is adopted, in order to convey more distinct ideas to the Faculty, and to place disorders of a similar nature nearest each other for their mutual illustration.

This was a reference to William Cullen's famous nosological classification of diseases. Haygarth was concerned that his old teacher should know of his studies. In the letter that Thomas Falconer had taken to Cullen in Edinburgh in 1772, he wrote,

---

[101] Corner and Booth, *Chain of Friendship*, 638.

[102] Assembly Book of the Chester Infirmary. Cheshire Record Office.

Mr Falconer will give you a plan for a register of births, &c, in Chester. You will observe that no distinctions are attempted but such as a parish clerk might understand. Any improvement that you would be so kind as to communicate, I shall be glad to adopt.[103]

Haygarth's work was gathered together in the paper that he later presented to the Royal Society in London. It was carried out with the meticulous care that he brought to all his future studies. His data were presented in a series of tables that contained the detailed information he had collected. The first table gave the number of deaths in the city by age and condition, each decade being considered separately. The next set out the diseases in detail, each age also being considered separately. There were columns for under 1, 1 to 2, 2 to 3, 3 to 5, 5 to 10, 10 to 15, and 15 to 20, then by decade until over 70. The diseases were classified as he had learned from Cullen into febrile (thirteen different causes), nervous (seven), diseases of habit (seven), and local diseases (seven). Tables III and IV dealt specifically with smallpox among the young, illustrating the seriousness of this disease as a cause of juvenile mortality. There were sixteen columns of inquiry setting out the population of the city parish by parish (there were ten parishes), comprising 3,428 families and a total population of 14,713. There were 625 individuals over the age of 70. Table VI gave the Bills of Mortality by parish and Table VII the deaths in each parish. This led him to the overall conclusion that the city of Chester was healthy, with a death rate of 1 in 40, a figure to be compared with that of other towns, such as Edinburgh (1 in 20 4/5), Manchester (1 in 28), Rome (1 in 23), and Amsterdam (1 in 24). Whites in Jamaica came off worst, with an appalling mortality rate of 1 in 5. Haygarth also made the irrelevant comment that "the women, especially in the higher and middle ranks of society, are remarkably beautiful."[104]

This work on disease in Chester was to be the basic framework upon which Haygarth built during his Chester years. As already noted, he was more fortunate in being able to study the city of Chester, with its relatively stable population, than were his colleagues working in urban conditions of overcrowding and shifting populations in cities such as Manchester or Liverpool. There, studies like Haygarth's, remarkable for their numerical accuracy, could not have been undertaken at that time.

[103]Thomson, *William Cullen,* 638.

[104]John Haygarth, "Observations on the Population and Diseases of Chester in the year 1774," *Philosophical Transactions of the Royal Society of London* 66 (1778): 151.

It was in this early paper that Haygarth gave the first hint of his plan to prevent the spread of fevers by isolation. A fever "which from its frequency might be called epidemical" (also called a malignant fever, possibly typhus) and smallpox had both been endemic during 1774. There were 285 cases of fever, with a mortality of 1 in 10. The proportion of smallpox deaths to all deaths had been 1 to 2 7/10, and out of a population of 14,713, only 1,060 (1 in 14) had never had smallpox. He particularly noted, as had his friend John Coakley Lettsom in London, that the highest mortality rate from fevers was among the poor, living in close, dirty habitations where fevers spread rapidly. His most radical suggestion was to advocate the immediate removal of people afflicted with fevers from their families, either into separate wards in the infirmary, which he thought might be objected to, or to a separate building on the grounds adjoining the infirmary. Haygarth's paper, "Observations on the Population and Diseases of Chester in the year 1774," was read to the Royal Society in London in November 1777. Curiously, there is no record of who arranged for this work to be presented to the prestigious Royal Society. Normally such work by a non-fellow would be presented on his behalf by a fellow, and this was the case for the papers presented at the same time as Haygarth's. William Heberden, who came to esteem his provincial colleague highly, is the most likely candidate for the role of Haygarth's supporter. He was at that time the medical member of the committee of the Royal Society that reviewed manuscripts before publication in *Philosophical Transactions*. There had been general dissatisfaction with the scientific standards of the society in the first half of the eighteenth century but in 1752, when the Earl of Macclesfield, a noted mathematician, was president, a committee had been set up to review all submissions. Haygarth's friend Thomas Percival, correspondent of William Heberden, was a fellow of the society and may well have played a part, as might have John Fothergill, who always shunned the limelight, and, as Lettsom put it, "was more desirous of doing good than of having it known."[105] Haygarth's paper was published in *Philosophical Transactions* the following year, presumably after perusal by Heberden. Two years later, in June 1780, John Haygarth of Chester, "Bachelor of Physic, formerly of St John's College, Cambridge, a gentleman of great merit and learning" was proposed as a fellow to the Royal Society, being "highly deserving of that honour & as he is likely to become a usefull & valuable member." He was duly elected

---

[105] J. C. Lettsom *Some Account of the Late John Fothergill, MD, FRS &c* (London: C. Dilly, 1784).

the following year. The first nominator was William Heberden, the second William Watson, and the third John Fothergill.[106]

By then, Heberden would have had good reason to know Haygarth. On November 11, 1773, Haygarth had given a paper at the College of Physicians, "A Case of the Angina Pectoris, with an attempt to investigate the Cause of the Disease by dissection, and a Hint suggested concerning the Method of Cure," which was published in the journal of the college.[107] Heberden had read his own original description of angina pectoris, a medical classic, to the college in 1768, but there were no dissections of his own patients and he had no idea that it was due to heart disease.[108] Haygarth's paper, therefore, although making no important discovery, must have been of some interest to Heberden, as it was one of the first in which a case was investigated by dissection after death. Heberden's 1768 paper had been published in 1772 in the first issue of *Medical Transactions of the College of Physicians of London*, of which he was himself an editor. It must have been he who vetted Haygarth's paper before its publication. Throughout his life Heberden remained a correspondent of Thomas Percival, and Heberden came to know Haygarth well. He wrote to Percival later in his life to tell him how long he had known and esteemed his Chester colleague.[109]

The cause of angina pectoris was soon to be greatly clarified by John Fothergill, who was the first to determine that it was a disorder of the heart when he described, with the aid of an autopsy carried out by John Hunter, calcified coronary arteries in angina pectoris.[110] John Fothergill was the founder of a small Society of Physicians in London that gathered at the Crown and Anchor in the Strand to read papers on matters of general concern. The proceedings were published, mostly at Fothergill's expense, in six volumes that appeared between 1752 and 1784. It must have been through Fothergill's influence that Haygarth read a paper to this society on January 12, 1778. He described a case of supposed hydrocephalus, outlining his

---

[106] Archives of the Royal Society, London. The other nominators were O. Brereton, G. Shuckburgh, William Steward, and Patrick Russell.

[107] John Haygarth, "A Case of the Angina Pectoris, with an attempt to investigate the Cause of the Disease by dissection, and a Hint suggested concerning the Method of Cure," *Medical Transactions of the College of Physicians of London* 3 (1785): 37–39.

[108] W. Heberden, "Some account of a disorder of the breast," *Medical Transactions of the College of Physicians of London* 2 (1772): 59–89.

[109] Heberden, *William Heberden,* 193.

[110] Christopher C. Booth, "Angina Pectoris and the Coronary Arteries," in Christopher C. Booth, *Doctors in Science and Society* (London: British Medical Journal, 1987), 84–94.

use of calomel in this and other cases. Although the results exceeded "my most sanguine expectations," he was cautious enough to warn that he could not with any confidence assert "that mercury in this case was the cause of recovery."[111]

[111] John Haygarth, "Apparent effect of Mercury in Cases that were supposed Hydrocephalus," *Medical Observations and Inquiries* 6 (1784): 58–67.

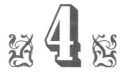

Smallpox and Other Infectious Fevers

Smallpox

*A*fter the mysterious disappearance of plague following the last great outbreak in England in 1665, smallpox became the most dreaded epidemic disease. In the words of Lord Macauley, it was "the most terrible of the ministers of death. . . . Smallpox was always present, filling the churchyards with corpses . . . and making the eyes and cheeks of the betrothed maiden objects of horror to the lover." It was smallpox that destroyed the Stuart dynasty and ensured the Hanoverian succession after the death of Queen Anne.

In Manchester, the smallpox epidemic of 1773 led Thomas Percival to the conclusion that mortality from smallpox had a vitally important impact on the country's rate of mortality. He recorded in detail the mortality rate from smallpox and the ages at which individuals succumbed to the disease, emphasizing the high mortality rate among young children. It is likely that Percival directed Haygarth's attention to the specific problem of epidemic smallpox among the young. He wrote later,

> My friend Dr Haygarth, to whom I had communicated the preceding *Tables of the comparative mortality of the smallpox* had adopted the plan and pursued the same inquiry at Chester. His statements will show how exactly our observations agree.[112]

---

[112] Cited in Lobo, "*John Haygarth*," 233.

Haygarth's findings were in fact very similar to those recorded by Percival. He had found, during the Chester epidemic that he recorded in his 1774 study, that the number of deaths from smallpox among children under 10 years of age was 369, compared with 736 from other diseases, illustrating how smallpox was then the prime cause of death among the young. These figures compared with death rates from smallpox in other cities that ranged from 1 in 6 to 1 in 9 deaths, figures very similar to those published for London earlier in the century by James Jurin, secretary to the Royal Society and physician to Guy's Hospital.[113] By 1777, Haygarth's observations on the mode of transmission had led him to the belief that although the usual method of transfer was contagion by immediate contact, there might be transmission of the infection through the air, but that this could only occur at a very short distance, less than a few feet from the infected person. At the same time, two circumstances made it particularly difficult to combat the infection. First were professional attitudes. Although by now few did not believe that smallpox was a contagious disease, there was still the waning medical belief that followed Sydenham in considering that infections became epidemic when there were atmospheric miasmata due to a morbid condition of the air. Haygarth dismissed such views with a blunt remark: "Whilst such an opinion prevails, the wildest visionary can never entertain a hope to retard the progress of this destructive malady [smallpox] except by prayers and the merciful interposition of Providence." Devout Anglican though he was, John Haygarth did not believe it was sufficient to trust in either providence or divine intervention. Second were the problems of popular fatalism. The poorer people did not hesitate to expose their children to smallpox—"to get it over with"—thereby encouraging the spread of the disease. At the same time, sufferers recovering from the disease but still infectious were walking on the city walls, in the streets, and in closes and rows, along with others who were susceptible to the disease. At that time very little thought had been given to the problem of how to prevent the spread of such diseases.

The Prevention of Smallpox

Haygarth's observations on the diseases of Chester, particularly smallpox, led him to suggest, first in private discussion with such local worthies as his friend Thomas Falconer, the formation of "The Smallpox Society." The

[113] Andrea A Rusnock, *The Correspondence of James Jurin (1684–1750)* (Amsterdam and Atlanta: Rodopi, 1996), 22–27.

idea of forming a society for a medical philanthropic purpose was not new. Lettsom, with whose work Haygarth was familiar through his discussions with Fothergill at Lea Hall, had founded a society of philanthropic gentlemen for the purpose of setting up the Dispensary at Aldersgate in 1770. But Haygarth's proposed society was the only one to be devoted to the prevention and eradication of a specific disease, a concept that only reached fruition in the twentieth century. The ideas that found practical expression in his Smallpox Society were put together by Haygarth as early as 1778, the year of his publication of the *Population and Diseases of Chester*, and he showed them that summer to Dr. Fothergill at Lea Hall. Benjamin Waterhouse, Fothergill's cousin from Rhode Island, was staying there that year. Haygarth must have been greatly encouraged by what Waterhouse told him. Until then, Haygarth did not know that "the smallpox had ever been excluded from any civilised country in the world." Waterhouse wrote from Lea Hall to Haygarth on September 25, 1778, "I have not forgot the promise I made to Dr Haygarth when we were last conversing upon the smallpox, of sending him an account of the means used in my native island, which so effectively secured us from the rage of that dreadful disease." Waterhouse described how, upon the recommendation of an appointed inspector, cases of smallpox were removed from their homes to a small island called Coastal Harbour. Initially this was done by removing the afflicted in a box big enough to house a small bed, but this was later changed to a sedan chair. If the disease was too far advanced for safe removal of the patient, the street in which the subject resided would be boarded up, guards placed, and the facts advertised in the local newspaper.[114]

Haygarth's concepts of smallpox were not published until 1784, yet they had been compiled several years earlier and circulated for comment to his correspondents, particularly his old teacher William Cullen.[115] As with so much that Haygarth published, his ideas were formulated as arguments and queries. He began with the obvious: Smallpox is an infective distemper that was never known to be produced by anything other than infection. He went on to argue that the variolous poison is soluble in air. Like a chemical substance added to water, it was entirely invisible. Unlike the dust particles that a sunbeam will reveal, smallpox miasmas cannot be seen. Furthermore, the poison is present in high concentration close to its origin from a smallpox patient, but becomes diluted farther away. The period between infection and

[114] John Haygarth, *An Inquiry How to Prevent the Smallpox* (London: J. Johnson; Chester: J. Monk, 1784), 138–146.

[115] Ibid.

commencement was six to fourteen days after inoculation and not much longer in natural smallpox. Persons liable to smallpox are infected, he argued, by breathing air impregnated with variolous miasma either very near to a smallpox patient or close to something containing the variolous poison. After various other arguments, Haygarth concluded that "the smallpox may be prevented by keeping Persons liable to the disorder from approaching within the infectious distance of the variolous poison."

Haygarth sent his proposed paper on variolous contagion to William Cullen in the summer of 1779. His respected teacher must have responded soon afterward, for Haygarth replied to him on September 11, 1779:

> I have taken your kind and judicious advice to study more attentively the nature of contagion, and with all the impartiality I could. Till I received the favour of your letter, I never read any account of the Plague except Sydenham, and one or two more imperfect than his. I have since carefully perused most of the books and passages that you pointed out, and was not a little pleased to find that they so amply confirmed some part of the doctrine I had endeavoured to establish in regard to the Small Pox.

But he wanted more advice. He went on,

> By the enclosed papers you will observe that further consideration of the subject has confirmed my former opinions, or, you might say prejudices. However, I have here more distinctly stated the chemical arguments which first suggested the thought, and cannot yet discover their fallacy. I entreat, as a very particular favour, that you would consider and rigidly criticise the arguments deduced, both from the chemical theory and the facts. . . . I shall expect with much anxiety your remarks on the enclosed papers, and particularly I request, as a *private* favour, your explicit answer to the queries at the conclusion.[116]

Yet the question that concerned Haygarth was not merely whether isolation procedures could prevent the spread of smallpox but whether the widespread practice of inoculation might be able to eradicate the disease.

Inoculation (variolation) is first documented in the Chinese literature, initially as a secret procedure dating from 1000 AD, but appearing in Chinese medical books by 1500. The mode of inoculation was by the intranasal insufflation of scab material from a patient with smallpox. There have been suggestions that variolation was practiced in India before European

---

[116] Thomson. *William Cullen*, 639–640.

settlement. In several European countries, including Wales, there were folk practices such as the seventeenth-century procedure of "buying the small-pox," in which children were sent to the homes of individuals recovering from smallpox to buy some crusts for a penny or two. In England during the eighteenth century, when, as Samuel Johnson remarked, there was a great passion for innovation, reports first appeared in 1700 describing the Chinese method of variolation by intranasal insufflation. Then, in 1714 and 1716, two independent accounts of the Turkish method of cutaneous in-oculation were communicated to the Royal Society in London by Emanuele Timoni and Jacob Pylarini.[117] At the same time, there was evidence that inoculation may have been practiced earlier in Africa. In 1716, during epidemics of smallpox in Boston, the Rev. Cotton Mather, notorious for his part in the witchcraft trials of Salem, learned of the practice from his African slave Onisemus.[118]

By the latter half of the eighteenth century, inoculation, which involved the inoculation into the skin of material from the pustule of a patient with smallpox, had become an established method for the prevention of the disease in England. The technique had been popularized by the remarkable Lady Mary Wortley Montagu, who as the wife of the British ambassador to the Turkish Sultan had had her son inoculated in Istanbul in 1718.[119] Inoculation had then received royal patronage when the future queen of George II, then Princess Caroline, had had her own children inoculated in 1722. Initially the practice, which produced a small crop of smallpox lesions around the site of inoculation, was not widely popular, as there were occasional fatalities. Furthermore, the inoculated individual could transmit the disease to the susceptible.

In the early years of the century, however, James Jurin, using his position as secretary of the Royal Society, played an important part in investigating whether smallpox induced by inoculation was safer than having the disease in the normal way. A mathematician by training as well as a physician, in 1722 he compared the Bills of Mortality from London and from colonial New England, where inoculation had been practiced since the year before.

---

[117] Emanuele Timoni, "An account or history of the procuring the smallpox by incision, or inoculation; as it has for some time been practiced at Constantinople." *Philosophical Transactions of the Royal Society of London* 29 (1714–1716): 72–82.

[118] Christopher C. Booth, "The Conquest of Smallpox," *Quarterly Journal of Medicine*, n.s. 57, 224 (1985): 811–823.

[119] Robert Halsband, *The Life of Lady Mary Wortley Montagu* (Oxford: Clarendon Press, 1956).

He was a pioneer in a century during which attempts were increasingly made to introduce quantitative methods into the problems of medical care.[120] He found that the hazard of inoculated smallpox was 1 in 49 or 50, whereas the risk of dying from the natural disease was as high as 1 in 7 or 8. There were other physicians, such as his friend, the distinguished physician and wit John Arbuthnot, who came to be convinced of the relative safety of the practice.[121] Remarkably, it was a provincial physician, Thomas Nettleton of Halifax in Yorkshire, who promoted further discussion, having learned of the procedure from Jurin's publication in the *Philosophical Transactions* of the Royal Society.[122] Jurin then went on to obtain accounts of the efficacy of inoculation from all parts of the country. Though Jurin did not practice inoculation himself, his position as secretary to the Royal Society enabled him to solicit information through the advertisement in the *Philosophical Transactions* in 1723 that had attracted the interest of Nettleton. Over sixty individuals sent accounts of their experience. Using this material, Jurin was able to publish annual reports on the use of the procedure by examining updated mortality figures.

Meanwhile, the London College of Physicians, in its customary leisurely fashion, did not publicly endorse the practice until 1755.[123] As the century wore on, inoculation became increasingly accepted after changes were made to the technique, particularly by the Suttons, sons of a surgeon in Debenham in Suffolk. They emphasized the importance of using one puncture only and the prescription of a spare diet, refrigerated drinks, and cool air. Quaker physician Thomas Dimsdale achieved fame, fortune, and his ennoblement as a baron by successfully inoculating the Empress Catherine of Russia and her children in 1767. He had been personally recommended to the Russian ambassador for this purpose by fellow Quaker John Fothergill.[124]

By the 1770s there had already been general inoculations in other cities throughout the land. Examples included Leeds, Liverpool, and Newcastle, as

---

[120] See Andrea A. Rusnock, *Vital Accounts: Quantifying Health and Population in Eighteenth-Century England and France* (Cambridge: Cambridge University Press, 2002).

[121] Rusnock, *James Jurin*, 23. See also Andrea A. Rusnock, "Biopolitics: Political Arithmetic in the Enlightenment," in *The Sciences in Enlightened Europe,* ed. William Clark, Jan Golinski, and Simon Schaffer (Chicago: University of Chicago Press, 1999).

[122] Ibid., 24.

[123] Annals of the Royal College of Physicians of London, vol. 12, folio 42, 22 December 1755.

[124] Fox, *Dr. Fothergill and His Friends,* 79–98. See also I. M. Gardner, "Two Hertfordshire Doctors," *Transactions of the East Hertfordshire Archeological Society* 13, pt. 1 (1952): 44–54.

well as West Hertfordshire in 1777, Luton in 1788, and Norfolk.[125] What made Haygarth's proposals different was his insistence on the "Rules of Prevention" that were to accompany inoculation. His rules were in fact a very practical implementation of his own views on how smallpox might be transmitted, namely that it could only pass from one person to another by direct contact or through the air over a very short distance. His rules were as follows:

RULES OF PREVENTION

1. Suffer no person, who has not had the smallpox, to come into an infectious house. No person who has had any communication with persons liable to the distemper, should touch or sit down on anything infectious.

2. No patient, after the pocks have appeared, must be suffered to go into the street, or other frequented place.

3. The utmost attention to *cleanliness* is absolutely necessary, *during* and *after* the distemper, no person, clothes, food, furniture, dog, cat, money, medicines, or any other thing that is known to be daubed with matter, spittle, or other infectious discharges of the patient, should go out of the house till they be washed, and till they have been sufficiently exposed to fresh air. No foul linen, or any thing else that can retain the poison, should be folded up and put into drawers, boxes, or be otherwise shut up from the air, but immediately thrown into water and kept there till washed. No attendants should touch what is to go into another family, till their hands are washed. When a patient dies of the smallpox, particular care should be taken that nothing infectious be taken out of the house so as to do mischief.

4. The patient must not be allowed to approach any person liable to the distemper, till every scab is dropt off, till all the clothes, furniture, food, and all other things touched by the patient during the distemper, till the floor of the sick chamber, and till his hair, face, and hands, have been carefully washed. After everything has been made perfectly clean, the doors, windows, drawers, boxes, and all other places that can retain infectious air should be kept open till it be cleared out of the house.

Haygarth made a habit of consulting his colleagues by correspondence and by setting out specific queries whenever he sought to publish the results of his studies. This led him to ask the following questions:

1. Do the rules of prevention contain an unnecessary restriction?

2. Do they comprehend every necessary restriction? Did you ever know three or more persons escape if certainly exposed?

---

[125] Peter Razzell, *The Conquest of Smallpox* (Firle, Sussex: Caliban Books, 1977).

3. Did you ever know of smallpox to be conveyed from one chamber into another by a person who did not carry any variolous serum or other infected matter?[126]

Presumably the responses to these queries were so self-evident that they simply confirmed Haygarth in what he had described to William Cullen as his prejudices. The respectful friendship that existed between Haygarth and his mentor was close, yet it came as a surprise to Haygarth that Cullen in his turn should choose to consult him on his own publications. When in late 1780 he received from Edinburgh the latest edition of Cullen's *Synopsis*, his wide-ranging classification of disease, he was greatly surprised that Cullen should ask him to transmit to him any remarks he might make on his *First Lines of the Practise of Physick*.[127] He replied,

I would not willingly disobey the commands of one to whom I owe so many, and such important, obligations. I wish rather to incur the censure of being presumptuous than ungrateful. But it should be remembered, that when we attempt to descry specks in the sun, we mean not dark but less luminous spots. Your candour, I trust, will excuse the humble hints submitted to your consideration with all possible deference. If they should contribute to render one tittle more perfect, a work that is likely to continue long instructing future physicians in our salutary science, I shall think my character as a critic well hazarded. I always highly admired your method of arranging diseases. But the last edition of your Synopsis greatly exceeded my expectation. It is a book that will be for ever in my hands, for I keep in concise Latin the cases of almost all my patients, and afterwards arrange them into genera according to your system.[128]

The Smallpox Society

The *Proceedings of the Society for Promoting of Inoculation at Stated Periods and Preventing of the Natural Smallpox in Chester* were published in 1784 by

[126] Haygarth. *Inquiry.* It should be stated here that some writers, for example Haygarth's biographer in the *DNB*, have referred to a publication by Haygarth of 1810 on the London pharmacopoeia. This is erroneous and derives from the binding together in the Library of the Royal College of Physicians of a copy of Haygarth's *Inquiry* with a copy of the *Pharmacopoeia Collegii Regalis*.

[127] William Cullen, *First Lines of the Practice of Physic* (Edinburgh: C. Eliot and London: T. Cadell, 1786).

[128] Thomson, *Life of Cullen*, 642.

Haygarth as an addendum to his *Inquiry How to Prevent the Smallpox*.[129] Haygarth must have had both enthusiasm and considerable influence among his fellow citizens to establish the Smallpox Society. He was much helped by his friend, the respected Chester citizen Thomas Falconer, who became chairman of the society and presided over its meetings. An advertisement was first put out on March 13, 1778, pointing out that 378 persons had died of smallpox in Chester during the past six years. Several of the magistrates and other respectable citizens had decided to call a public meeting at the Pentice, one of Chester's ancient courts, named for its having been established in the penthouse of a medieval building. This was to take place on Monday, March 16, at 11 o'clock in the morning, in order to set up the society. It was clearly a philanthropic venture, aimed at relieving the calamity of smallpox that fell "upon the poor and greatly aggravated their complicated wretchedness." As to financing the proposal, it was pointed out that "the *moderate* contribution of the *many* would fix the Society on the firmest foundation." Charges were to include 5 shillings for an inoculation and rewards of 2 shillings were to be given to compliant parents. A contribution of 1 guinea would entitle a subscriber to recommend three persons to be inoculated, and 10 guineas would secure that right for life. Physicians were to give their services gratis. There were also to be inspectors who reported on the faithful following of the regulations as well as recommending rewards and giving certificates.

Meetings of the society were held at the Pentice for the next four years. By February 1780, there were 149 members of the society, including as medical members the Chester physicians Drs. Denton, Haygarth, and Currie as well as six apothecaries and surgeons. The last meeting took place on September 17, 1782, when the company concluded, "Our united example and influence might prove of great importance to our country and to mankind." At that meeting the society's cumulated accounts were published. It had been a viable venture. Receipts had amounted to £199:2:6 and expenditure was £170:3:0. In later years, Haygarth recorded that the society had existed for six years and then only ceased because the poor people refused to accept gratuitous inoculation of their children.

The reports of the society were written by Haygarth. At first it seemed that the plan was working well. The number of deaths from casual smallpox in Chester declined by half while the society operated. At the end of the first twelve months, the disease was stopped in thirty-seven places, in thirty-two of these without affecting another family. Inoculations were

[129] Haygarth, *Inquiry.*

repeated each year, with only 2 fatalities in 416 inoculations. But parents increasingly resisted inoculation for their children and there were difficulties in ensuring that the "Rules for Prevention" were adhered to. In particular, irresponsible soldiery on their way to service in Ireland and wandering on the city walls might spread the disease. The overall results, however, were so striking that Leeds and Liverpool followed Chester's example. Countries in certain parts of Europe were equally interested in the Chester experience after the reports of the society were published along with Haygarth's *An Inquiry How to Prevent the Smallpox* in 1784. It was translated into French and German and in 1791 Haygarth was asked to advise the Syndick and Council of Geneva on the establishment of a similar institution. A copy of his book is preserved in the library of the Royal College of Physicians, with an inscription in his own hand, "For Dr Currie," presumably William Currie, his Chester colleague who had labored with him in the Smallpox Society.

Haygarth's Manchester friend, Thomas Percival, was one of those who enthusiastically supported the *Enquiry*. He wrote to his friend,

> I most cordially rejoice that your very benevolent and judicious *Inquiry how to prevent the Small Pox*, has already excited and is still more likely to excite, the attention and approbation of the public; and I admire the steadiness and zeal with which you have prosecuted this plan. . . . I shall feel a pride and a pleasure in contributing in any way towards the accomplishment of your laudable views. . . . I shall be happy in the opportunity of conferring with you at Warrington on these and other interesting topics.[130]

But he had another project in mind. He thought that Haygarth should ensure that the empress of Russia—a great woman possessed of both enterprise and the power to carry her desires into effect—should receive a French translation of the work. If Haygarth had no connections with St. Petersburg, Dr. Rogerson, first physician to the empress, had recently visited him and he would arrange for him to present the book. There is no evidence that this ever happened.

Like James Jurin before him, Haygarth, unusually for those days, was a pioneer in the use of mathematical analysis in clinical research, a reflection no doubt of his schooling with John Dawson at Sedbergh. In his publication, Haygarth set out the arithmetical calculations made by "a mathematical friend," almost certainly Dawson, on the degree of possibility of escaping

---

[130] Percival, *Memoirs,* cix.

smallpox when exposed for the first time to the disorder. Dawson, if it was he, made the following computation:

> If there be one person in 20 who is not liable to the smallpox, it is therefore evident that, for any particular person, there are 19 chances that he may be infected, and only one that he may not. Hence we may reason, however epidemical the smallpox has been in a town, that a child who has escaped the distemper, was never exposed to the infection (unless we know to the contrary) is probable in a degree of 19 to one. If two in a family have escaped, the probability that they were never both exposed is above 400 to one: if three in a family escapes, above 8000 to one.[131]

Influenza

Haygarth had a wide-ranging mind that did not restrict itself to the problem of smallpox that had so engrossed him during those years.[132] He was also interested in other infectious diseases and on two occasions took part in national investigations of epidemic influenza. There had been a widespread epidemic of the disease in England and Ireland in 1775, and from London Fothergill had undertaken, with the help of friends and colleagues, the conduct of a nationwide survey. He wrote to a number of respected colleagues, among them Sir John Pringle, William Heberden, and Sir George Baker inquiring as to their experience of the disorder. His correspondents also included his old friend and fellow student in Edinburgh, William Cuming of Dorchester, Dr. Ash in Birmingham, and others as far afield as Lancaster and Aberdeen. Haygarth replied from Chester that in a street of affluent residents, 73 out of 97 suffered; in one of tradespeople, 109 out of 114; and in the home of industry 175 occupants had been affected. Bleeding and the bark [chinchona bark from South America, a source of quinine] were often used in treatment. Haygarth advised "*Tartar emetic gr ¼, 2 dis. Horis as sursum vel dorsum purgandum.*"[133]

[131] Haygarth, *Inquiry*, 27.

[132] For influenza in the eighteenth century, see Margaret De Lacy, "Influenza Research and the Medical Profession in Eighteenth Century Britain," *Albion* 25 (1993): 37–66; Margaret De Lacy, "The Conceptualisation of Influenza in Eighteenth Century Britain: Specificity and Contagion," *Bulletin of the History of Medicine* 67 (1993): 74–118.

[133] John Fothergill, "A Sketch of the Epidemic Disease which appeared in London towards the end of the year 1775," in *The Works of John Fothergill M. D.*, ed. J. C. Lettsom (London: Charles Dilly, 1784), 615–643.

By the time of the 1782 epidemic, Fothergill was dead, and this time it was the College of Physicians in London that conducted the survey. The college sent a questionnaire to physicians throughout the land to inquire about their experience of the disease. Haygarth, although as a provincial physician never a fellow of the college, was one of those consulted and his observations were communicated to the college by his friend William Heberden. In his carefully written document of nearly thirty pages,[134] accompanied by a letter to the registrar of the college, Dr. Henry Revell Reynolds,[135] Haygarth described where the first cases occurred in Chester and its surrounding villages, at which dates (in particular in comparison with other areas of the country), and how long the disorder might last. His report includes responses to his queries addressed to many neighboring physicians. It became clear to him that influenza generally started in large towns, spread to other smaller places, and only later would appear in more isolated places and surrounding villages. In 1775, for example, the disease reached Chester about the middle of November, the first patient having been the landlady of one of the principal inns of the city. In the neighboring villages, however, the disease did not appear until some ten days later. As to its origin, Haygarth quoted from *Sketch of the Epidemic* of 1775, written by his "highly respected friend, Dr Fothergill." The disease then appeared to have spread from London "about the beginning of November, that is, near a fortnight earlier than in Chester." The movement and spread of the malady was well attested by "curious and instructive intelligence from my ingenious friend Dr Dobson who at that time resided in Liverpool."[135] As to the influenza of 1775, he found that it prevailed along the coast of the Mediterranean in September but was almost over by the beginning of November. It reached England, however, in early November but did not ever appear in the West Indies, the continent of America, Sweden, Denmark, or the more northern parts of Europe. Haygarth noted one other remarkable fact: None of his inpatients in the infirmary contracted the disease.

Haygarth's account of the influenza epidemic in 1782 bore out his previous observations of 1775 and in this section of his paper he characteristically

[134] John Haygarth, "Of the manner in which the Influenza spread in Chester and its neighbourhood in 1775 and 1782," report to the College of Physicians communicated by William Heberden MD, fellow of the College and of the Royal Society, Library of the Royal College of Physicians of London. Accompanied by autograph letter to Dr. Reynolds.

[135] Henry Revell Reynolds (1745–1811) was registrar of the College of Physicians from 1781 to 1783 and later a physician to George III. William Munk, *Roll of the Royal College of Physicians of London* (London: The College, Pall Mall East, 1888), 2:299–301.

included a detailed table showing the first dates of appearance of the disease in Chester and the surrounding countryside. He clearly showed how, as in 1775, the disease spread from Chester itself to the smaller towns and villages around the city. As was his usual practice in dealing with medical problems, Haygarth posed a series of questions before reaching his conclusions.

"Is the Influenza conveyed from one place to another like the wind?" he asked, "or does it spread through the atmosphere like sound, or like a wave made by a pebble thrown into a smooth surface of water [this sentence was crossed out], from a centre gradually & uniformly to all the surrounding places?" Either of these suppositions was in his view fully refuted. He then asked whether the first patient coming into a town "contaminates the atmosphere of the place so as to render it generally pestilential in regard to this distemper? If this hypothesis were true, I should expect the seizure to have been much more general and sudden than actually took place," a clear refutation that the disorder might be transmitted by atmospheric miasmata. He considered whether "climate, wind or season" might determine propagation but found no evidence to support any of these factors. His final question, which was really his conclusion after careful argument and consideration, was, "Is the influenza spread by the infection of patients in the Distemper?" Although he cautiously wrote that the proofs were not yet in his view complete, he considered that "these facts afford some presumption that the Distemper was propagated by personal infection." In other words, like smallpox, the disease was spread by person-to-person contact. Yet there was one major difference: The interval between exposure and development of influenza was very much shorter than in smallpox.[134]

Infectious Disease in Farm Animals

The problem of infectious disease among cattle and other farm animals must have been very familiar to anyone brought up in the rural environment of Garsdale. Haygarth in particular, must have been concerned that the rules that governed the transmission of infectious disease in humans were equally applicable to animals. There is tantalizingly little evidence of Haygarth's views, with the exception of a fragment preserved in the Chester Record Office. Among other documents relating to Dr. Haygarth is a paper in his characteristic handwriting. It sets out, as was so usual with Haygarth, a series of queries relating to the transmission of an infection among animals:

Was Francis Kinsey's cow of Melborne the first seized in the neighbourhood.

Is Kinsey a mere farmer or has he any connection with any tanner, or business that employs any hides or hair of cows.

What distance is he from any wharf where any hides or other goods are imported from Holland or the Baltick.

Is he a carrier from such wharf or could his cows be exposed to infection contained in straw or other package of goods imported from abroad.

Is it well ascertained that the pigs at Challerton smelt & li[c]ked the head of Kinsey's cow & soon afterwards died?

Is the distemper entirely stopt

Are all infected cows killed as soon as they are known to be attacked, and buried, their hides being previously slashed.[136]

These queries, posed in Haygarth's characteristic manner, indicate that he took an interest in the infectious diseases of animals, but there is no evidence in any of his other writings that he was involved in veterinary matters.

[136] Manuscript fragment, unsigned, in the handwriting of John Haygarth, Cheshire Record Office.

From Fever Wards to Fever Hospitals

The Establishment of Fever Wards at the Chester Infirmary

*F*or any lesser man it might be imagined that the demise of the smallpox so-ciety would represent a setback. For John Haygarth, however, whose mind was ever fertile, there were two questions that were raised by his experiences thus far. The first was his ever-present concern with the prevention of smallpox, a subject that continued to consume his interest and to which he was to return a decade later. The second was how to deal with the more general problem of fever in the community that he served. In London, the establishment by Lett-som of the dispensaries had provided medical care for fever among the poor, who had no access to the London hospitals, in their own homes.[137] But there was no emphasis in London on how the spread of fever could be prevented. In fact, the London dispensaries were staffed by men who had no connection with the London hospitals, mostly dissenters debarred from the fellowship of the Royal College of Physicians. There was therefore no way in which they could have persuaded the hospitals to interest themselves in the control of fever. Hay-garth in Chester was in a different position. Not only was he a physician to the infirmary but he was also by now a figure of some significance in Chester society. It was perhaps for these reasons that he was able to achieve a degree of success in the control of fever that was denied to his colleagues in the metropo-lis. In later years, however, they were to follow his example.

[137] Robert Kirkpatrick, 'Living in the Light.' Dispensaries, philanthropy and medical reform in late-eighteenth-century London. In: *The Medical Enlightenment of the Eighteenth Century*, ed. Andrew Cunningham and Roger French (Cambridge: Cambridge University Press, 1990).

By 1780–1781, having shown that the infectivity of smallpox was limited to a short distance from the patient, he turned his attention to the spread of febrile conditions in general. He had learned from William Cullen that certain fevers, for example jail or hospital fever, were, like smallpox, spread by contagion, and he thought that, as with smallpox, their infectivity was limited to a short distance. He had proposed as early as 1774 that it would be advantageous to admit fever patients to a separate building on the grounds of the hospital, but he now thought it both safe and wise to admit such patients to separate wards in the Chester Infirmary. He was not the first to propose such measures, for James Lind, working as a naval surgeon at the Haslar Hospital in the 1760s, had concluded that the common ship fevers that so frequently afflicted sailors were contagious. He attempted to counter their transmission by strict measures of isolation and by burning infected clothing. He also fumigated the wards with brimstone, tobacco, or gunpowder. At the same time, he introduced separate fever wards in the hospital, just as Haygarth was to do twenty years later in Chester.[138] It was, however, one thing for a medical officer in a naval hospital to achieve his aims by edict. It was quite another for a civilian physician, working in a community where concepts of miasma led people to think that fever would spread through the atmosphere, to persuade his colleagues that the establishment of such wards was the right approach. Haygarth's proposals, furthermore, were far more ambitious than Lind's. He was essentially setting out to influence the public health of his city. By ensuring that patients with fever would be removed from their families to wards where they would be cared for, he not only ensured that they would receive medical attention but also sought to prevent the spread of fever.

In 1783, Chester was alarmed by an epidemic of fever. In particular there was an extension of cases of fever, sometimes fatal, from their customary haunt in the poverty-stricken hovels of the poor to the homes of the higher echelons of Chester society. Haygarth took the opportunity to put his ideas into effect and immediately sought suitable accommodation for the effective isolation of cases of fever.[139] He soon found that in the attic story of the infirmary there was an unoccupied space, 96 feet long and 21 feet wide, that was open to the roof and divided by a partition. The ventilation was good, there was a room for a nurse, and there was "a separate necessity

[138] Ulrich Trohler, *To Improve the Evidence of Medicine* (Edinburgh: Royal College of Physicians of Edinburgh, 2000), 29.

[139] John Haygarth, *A Letter to Dr Percival on the Prevention of Infectious Fevers* (Bath: R. Crutwell, 1801).

which prevented personal intercourse with the rest of the hospital." There were difficulties at first in obtaining nurses for the new wards, such was the fear of contracting fever from the patients. The first nurse was a male surgical patient, who did in fact succumb. The next was Lowry Thomas, who cared for the fever patients for eleven years. She contracted fever several times and finally died of an attack in 1794. She was succeeded by Jane Bird. Both of these courageous and pioneering nursing colleagues should be remembered in any Valhalla of medical fame.

The fever wards were a success from the start. The transmission of fevers in the city was effectively arrested and at the same time fever did not spread elsewhere in the hospital, as some had feared that it might. By 1796, Haygarth was able to report to his friend Thomas Percival in Manchester, telling him that during twelve years of operation of the fever wards "it had never been suspected that the patients in other parts of the house have caught any Infection from the Fever Wards by any contamination of the atmosphere." Haygarth concluded at that time that "our fever wards do ten times more good in the prevention of misery and the preservation of life than all the other parts of the Infirmary."[140]

It may well be asked what the views were of the denizens of the hovels of the poor who were admitted to the fever wards. There is no evidence; many were illiterate and left no record of their experiences. For those who supported the charitable foundations of those days, it was generally considered that hospitals were "mirrors of godliness."[141] Charity, it has been argued, "was a way for the rich to buy salvation."[142] But, as in Chester, there were other motives that were entirely altruistic. In the later years of the eighteenth century, charity thrived. By 1760, trusts had doubled since the beginning of the century, and thirty years later the total amount raised was as much as £250,000.[143]

It has been suggested that the charity hospitals in England had a bad reputation as death traps. While this may have been true on the continent of Europe, where, in Aix-en-Provence for example, entry to a hospital was regarded as a last resort, so the poor would do anything to avoid admission, this does not seem to have been the case in England. In eighteenth-

[140] Ibid., 3.

[141] Mary E. Fissell, *Patients, Power and the Poor in Eighteenth Century Bristol* (Cambridge: Cambridge University Press, 1991).

[142] Cissie C. Fairchilds, *Poverty and Charities in Aix-en-Provence* (Baltimore: Johns Hopkins Press, 1976).

[143] Anne Borsay, *Medicine and Charity in Georgian Bath: A Social History of the General Infirmary. 1739–1830* (Aldershot: Ashgate, 1999).

century Bristol, Mary Fissell has shown that the hospital was much in demand and the death rate was not much more than 4 percent, even though fever patients were freely admitted, making up as many as 16 percent of total admissions. There were, however, concerns among paupers, whose bodies might be handed to the anatomists for dissection. Richard Smith, surgeon to the infirmary and friend of John Haygarth during his years in Bath, was an enthusiastic dissector. In fact, in Bath there is no evidence that patients regarded the infirmary as anything other than a haven in times of affliction. In Chester, Haygarth did not hesitate, in his reports of the Smallpox Society, to describe the opposition of poor people to having their children inoculated. There is, by contrast, no suggestion in his writings that there was any significant opposition among his patients to the fever wards in Chester.

As far as the wider world was concerned, there were few, other than Haygarth's friends and medical correspondents, who were aware of what was happening in Chester. John Howard, however, Quaker philanthropist and prison reformer, visited Chester in 1788.[144] Born in 1726, Howard was a close friend of John Fothergill. Despite being a dissenter, he was appointed high sheriff of Bedfordshire in 1773 and was at once shocked by the state of the prisoners in the local jails and bridewells. In particular he was concerned with the depredations of jail fever and smallpox among prisoners, as well as the practice of keeping those not guilty in jail until they had paid a fee to the jailer. In London at the same time Fothergill had given evidence with Howard to the House of Commons that led to the passing of an act for preserving the health of prisoners in jail. Later, Howard and Fothergill were to be involved together in government plans for the erection of better penitentiary houses. Howard had made his first visitations to the prisons in England and Wales in 1775 and had published his experiences in his *State of the Prisons* two years later, when he had moved to Warrington. His visit to Chester in 1788 was undertaken during his fourth and last nationwide survey. He must have been well known to John Haygarth, who seized the opportunity to show him what was going on in the Chester Infirmary and in the local schools.

Howard was not overly impressed by the Chester prisons but he made a particular point of commenting favorably on the fever wards of the Chester Infirmary. He pointed out that Dr. Haygarth and his colleagues had set up the wards in response to the depredations of the contagious fever in Chester in 1784, when most of the patients had recovered. He commented, "The

---

[144] John Howard (1726?–1790), *Oxford DNB;* 28:390–394.

wards are spacious and clean, and the beds not crowded. The two fever wards wcrc not in the least offensive." He then copied the "good rules" for the fever wards, which were clearly adapted from Haygarth's rules of prevention for the control of smallpox. Because they laid the foundation for the way fever wards would be run during the next century, they deserve to be printed in full:

> *Rules for the Fever Wards; to prevent the Infection of other Patients in the Chester Infirmary*
>
> *Chester Infirmary Rules.*—I. Fresh water and coals are to be brought up to the fever wards every morning; and other necessaries on ringing a bell.
>
> II. No fever patients, nor their nurses are suffered to go into other parts of the house. No other patient is allowed to visit the Fever Wards; nor any stranger, unless accompanied by the apothecary or his assistant.
>
> III. Every patient, on admission, is to change his infectious for clean linen; the face and hands are to be washed clean with warm water, and the lower extremities fomented.
>
> IV. All putrid discharges from the patient are to be taken out of the ward as soon as possible.
>
> V. The floors of the wards are to be washed very clean twice a week, and near the beds every day.
>
> VI. All foul linen is to be immediately thrown into cold water; and carefully washed twice out of clean water, in the adjoining room.
>
> VII. Blankets, and other bed and body clothes are to be exposed to the open fresh air for some hours, before they are used by another patient.
>
> VIII. All the bed clothes of the fever wards are to be marked "FEVER WARD", and all the knives, forks, pots, cups, and other utensils are to be of a peculiar colour, lest they be inadvertently taken among other patients.
>
> IX. All the windows of the fever wards are to be kept constantly open in the day, except the weather be very cold or wet; and some of them should not be shut in the night, if the patients be numerous, and the weather moderate.
>
> X. No relation or other acquaintance can be suffered to take away any linen unwashed, nor other clothes till they have been exposed to the fresh air.[145]

---

[145] John Howard, *An Account of the Principal Lazarettos in Europe: with various papers relating to the Plague: together with further Observations on some Foreign Prisons and Hospitals* (Warrington: W. Eyres and London: T. Cadell, 1789), 208–209.

The Fever Hospital Movement

The concept of isolation in the prevention of the spread of infectious disease was not new: The lazarettos of the Mediterranean ports had sought to prevent the entry of plague, and hospitals for smallpox were commonplace. What was new was the idea that the isolation of patients suffering from the common forms of fever and their removal from the community would prevent them from infecting others. Haygarth's ideas soon spread to other centers, particularly through the influence of the many medical friends with whom he kept in close contact. In Birmingham, his fellow Edinburgh student, William Withering, applied Haygarth's method of isolation to the management of scarlet fever, a more severe affliction then than in our own time. Withering wrote, "From the time that Dr Haygarth first communicated to me his ideas for stopping the progress of smallpox, the probability of stopping the progress of Scarlet Fever by similar methods was too evident to escape the most attentive observer. . . . And now for several years past I have never thought it necessary to break up a private school, or to disperse a private family."[146]

In Manchester, Haygarth's close friend Thomas Percival was an influential figure. He joined the staff of the Manchester Infirmary in 1780 and was at once involved in attempts to improve the health care available to the poor. Unlike the situation in London, where dispensaries were increasingly important in the provision of succor to the disadvantaged, there was no dispensary in Manchester. Instead, uniquely in England, Manchester developed a dispensary service built onto the existing work of the infirmary.[147] In 1781, a home-patient service was introduced by the assistant physicians. As in the dispensaries that followed Lettsom's London model, patients were seen as outpatients and could also be both seen and treated at home. Although fever patients could now receive attention, both the infirmary and the local workhouses refused admission to fever patients, as was the case in London and elsewhere. In the middle of the 1790s, when economic stagnation and hard winters led to grain shortages and an exacerbation of poverty, outbreaks of fever became increasingly common in Manchester. By now the physicians to

---

[146]William Withering, *An Account of the Scarlet Fever and Sore Throat or Scarlatina Anginosa. Particularly as it appeared at Birmingham in the year 1779* (London: T. Cadell, 1799).

[147] Pickstone, *Medicine and Industrial Society.* For further information on the House of Recovery in Manchester, see Frank Renaud, *A Short History of the House of Recovery or Fever Hospital in Manchester* (Manchester: Cornish, 1885).

the infirmary, led by Percival and John Ferrier, were pressing for the establishment of a hospital for fever patients. The municipal authorities, alarmed at the number of fever patients, which was reaching epidemic proportions, were equally concerned. Armed with the opinions of their medical friends, particularly John Haygarth, the Manchester physicians prepared a paper setting out their views, emphasizing Haygarth's contention that patients were only infectious to a very short distance and that the spread of infection could therefore be prevented by isolation. In 1794, the Manchester board of health published an extract of a letter to Dr. Percival from Haygarth, who wrote from Chester,

> A typhous Fever became very epidemical among the poor in Chester, about the time it began in Manchester; our Fever wards in the Infirmary became crowded to a greater degree than they have been since the establishment of this regulation, near a dozen years ago. But these measures have checked the progress of the epidemick; very few patients are now heard of in the whole town. The regulations proposed by your physicians will undoubtedly be of service; but, in my opinion, are quite inadequate to cure the malady. A Fever Hospital annexed to your Infirmary, to hold about twenty patients of each sex, would save a multitude of lives in your populous town. Your physicians who visit the home-patients, are exposed to imminent danger of contagion; in a well-ventilated, clean hospital, the medical attendant is not, I apprehend, liable to infection. I am, and have been for several years, collecting facts to illustrate various questions relative to this interesting subject.[148]

The fever hospital in Manchester, however, was not established without a struggle. Local residents objected, claiming that neighboring inhabitants would be put at risk. There were also questions as to what the hospital should be called. Finally the name House of Recovery was agreed to, an inspired choice, and it was opened in May 1796. The benefit appears to have been immediate. The number of fever cases in Manchester fell from 267 during the first year to 25 in the next. At the same time, the Bills of Mortality showed a decrease in the number of burials of nearly 400. The civic authorities were also gratified that the expense of pauper coffins was reduced by a third.

In Liverpool, James Currie was an influential figure in pressing for improvements in the provision of health care to the poor. Like Lettsom in London, he had considerable experience of the appalling conditions in which the

---

[148] Haygarth, *Letter to Dr Percival*, 3.

poor lived from his work at the Liverpool Dispensary. He also had a particular interest in the treatment of fevers. He had introduced the technique of cold douches for the treatment of fevers and had been the first in Britain to use a clinical thermometer to assess their efficacy. Currie was a close friend of Haygarth, a member of the group that met regularly in Warrington, and he knew of the pioneering work in Chester. It was therefore not surprising that in Liverpool it was Currie who pressed for the establishment of a fever hospital. For five years, from 1796 to 1801, and against strong opposition, Currie carried on the fight to receive the poor in the hospital when suffering from infectious disease. He wrote,

> To pronounce a disease to be contagious, ought not to deprive the sufferer of the aids of science or of humanity, as some weakly suppose. It ought now to be generally known, that simple means of precaution, *adopted early and strictly adhered to,* do away the danger to the attendants; and the practitioner of medicine who cannot trust his own safety to those, is unworthy of his office, and ought to lay it down.[149]

It was not to be achieved in his lifetime. Building of the Liverpool House of Recovery was begun in 1801 but it was not opened until 1806.[147] Currie had died the previous year.

London, the metropolis where Lettsom had played so important a role in founding the first general dispensary in 1770, lagged behind other urban centers in its provision of care for patients with fever. But there were friends of Haygarth in the capital who sought to follow his example. At Guy's Hospital, William Saunders (1743–1817)[150] pressed for the allocation of two wards as fever wards, and at St. George's, William Heberden, longtime admirer of his provincial colleague, knew that money was becoming available for development. It was he who suggested that resources should be set aside for the provision of fever wards. At the same time, both Lettsom and dermatologist Robert Willan, physician to the Carey Street Dispensary, gave strong support to the idea of a fever hospital for London. It was not, however, until 1801 that London's citizens began to stir themselves.[151] As

[149] R. D. Thornton, *James Currie, The Entire Stranger and Robert Burns* (Edinburgh and London: Oliver and Boyd, 1963).

[150] William Saunders (1743–1813), *Oxford DNB; 49:51–52.*

[151] W. F. Bynum, "Hospital, Disease and Community: The London Fever Hospital, 1801–1850," in *Healing and History: Essays for George Rosen,* ed. Charles E. Rosenberg (London: Dawson, Science History Publications, 1979).

elsewhere, it was local epidemics of fever in the capital that provided the spur. Lettsom was one of the moving spirits. He had written extensively that same year on the prevention of infectious fevers in his *Hints Designed to Promote Beneficence, Temperance and Medical Science*, emphasizing the importance of isolation. He particularly praised his Chester friend, John Haygarth, writing,

> However obvious these facts must appear, and however easy the means of stopping the progress of infection must prove, adequate attention has not been paid to these subjects, in any large town, within these realms, until my learned and humane friend, Dr Haygarth . . . of Chester, suggested a plan, and carried it into effect in the City of Chester, for preventing and stopping the progress of infectious fevers.[152]

The London Fever Hospital was launched on May Day 1801. The founders were predominantly laymen but at that first meeting a letter from fifteen London physicians was read. The signatories were mainly men from the London hospitals but also included Robert Willan and Thomas Murray, both from the Carey Street Dispensary and therefore men well versed in the problems of fever among the poor. Willan in particular had written extensively on the condition of the poor in London. The fever hospital letter would have had Haygarth's enthusiastic support. He could almost have written it himself. It read as follows:

> Having been desired to state our sentiments on the situation of the Poor with respect to Contagion, we declare that Infectious, Malignant Fever is at all times prevalent among the Poor of the Metropolis, in whose habitations it has an instant tendency to diffuse itself more widely; that it often extends from them to the higher orders; that it derives its origin principally from neglect of cleanliness and ventilation; and that its communication from the first person attacked, to the other members of a family is an almost necessary consequence of the crowded state of the dwellings of the Poor. . . . We believe that in many instances the infection of a family and neighbourhood is owing to contagion introduced by a single person, and would be prevented by his timely removal. We are therefore satisfied that the evils above mentioned would be in great measure obviated by the establishment of an institution which should have for its object—the removal of persons attacked by Contagious Fever from situations where, if they remain, the infection of others is inevitable.[151]

---

[152] John Coakley Lettsom, *Hints Designed to Promote Beneficence, Temperance and Medical Science* (London: J. Nichols, 1801).

The London Fever Hospital was to have a distinguished history, only to merge with the Royal Free Hospital Group at the advent of the National Health Service in 1948. Many other cities adopted the regulations that had been formulated by Haygarth at Chester. By the end of the first decade of the nineteenth century Haygarth could record that Edinburgh, Newcastle, Leeds, Dublin, Waterford, and Cork had followed the Chester example. "The measures have now been proved, by extensive experience," he wrote, "to be so practicable, and so completely successful for the prevention of infectious Distempers, that the example will probably be followed in all large towns."[153]

[153] Haygarth, *Letter to Dr Percival*, 3.

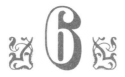

Other Activities in Chester

The Blue-Coat School: The Education of the Children of the Poor

*I*n his travels around the kingdom, John Howard was interested not only in prisons but also in the schools that he encountered. In Chester, John Haygarth had taken the opportunity of showing him the fever wards at the Chester Infirmary of which he was so proud, but at the same time he made sure that Howard knew what Chester was doing to provide for the education of the children of the poor. Haygarth, in his studies of the population of Chester and his attempts to wipe out smallpox, had good reason for understanding the relationship between ignorance and disease. He shared the views of John Locke, who had written, "Of all the men we meet with, nine parts of ten are what they are, good or evil, useful or not, by their Education. It is that which makes the great difference among mankind."[154] He also believed, as did John Howard, that the prevalence of crime in any area was directly related to the quality of education available. "Ignorance," he wrote, "is the parent of vice." His friend, Archibald Maclaine (1722–1804),[155] the chaplain to the British embassy in Holland who had retired to Bath in 1796, told him that in the United Provinces all the natives, even the lowest, were taught to read and write, and some of them were instructed in arithmetic. In The Hague, where Dr. Maclaine had lived for half a century, not a single

---

[154] John Locke, *Some Thoughts Concerning Education,* ed. with introduction, notes, and critical apparatus by John W. Yolton and Jean S. Yolton, the Clarendon Edition of the Works of John Locke (Oxford: Clarendon Press, 1989).

[155] Archibald Maclaine (1722–1804), a native of Monaghan, was the son of Lachlan Maclaine and brother of the notorious highwayman James Maclaine, who was hanged at Tyburn in 1750. He was originally assistant to his maternal uncle, Robert Milling, pastor of the English church in The Hague. He moved to Bath in 1796, where presumably he came to meet John Haygarth. See *Oxford DNB,* 35:716–717.

native of that town of 40,000 inhabitants had been executed for any crime during that whole time. Haygarth was also able to state that in the area of the northwest of England where he was brought up and educated there was a similar lack of major crime, which he equated with the educational facilities available, particularly at his own school at Sedbergh.[156]

In Chester, the Blue-Coat School had been founded as a charity in 1700 and the school that Haygarth came to know was built in 1717. Blue-Coat schools had originated in Tudor times; Christ's Hospital in London was the first. The name derives from the long blue coats worn by pupils, to which were added in later years the characteristic yellow stockings and white collars. Blue was originally chosen because it was the cheapest dye available at the time. The schools spread during the next two centuries, so that by the beginning of the eighteenth century there were perhaps sixty Blue-Coat schools in England. As in other towns throughout the kingdom, the Chester Blue-Coat School was maintained by the charitable contributions of the more opulent and beneficient inhabitants, who hence became Trustees. Haygarth himself was a trustee for many years, as was Thomas Falconer. It was due to Haygarth's efforts that the school was to play an important part in the education of the poor of the city. In 1780, there were thirty boys who were educated and maintained at the school. They were boarders, and there were no day boys. At that time there was an increase in the money available to the trustees and the proposal was made that the number of boys should be increased by five. In 1783, however, Haygarth ventured a proposal to extend the benefit of instruction to a much larger number of children. He suggested that the boys should remain "in-scholars" for two instead of four years, and that instead of five additional in-scholars, there should be 120 "out-scholars" (effectively day boys) who would be taught to read, write, and manage some arithmetic. These out-scholars were to be provided with green caps, at a cost of 1 shilling and 6 pence, so they became known as "green-caps." He also proposed that after two years, fifteen of the out-scholars who had been the most diligent and were the most proficient should be selected by the trustees, after due examination, to supply the in-scholar vacancies at the school, where they would be maintained for two more years. Haygarth was able to calculate from his own studies of the population that 120 out-scholars and

---

[156] John Haygarth's endeavors in reorganizing the activities of the Blue-Coat School in Chester were not published until 1812, when he included his own account in *A Private Letter addressed to the Right Reverend Dr Porteus, the Lord Bishop of London, to Propose a Plan, which might give a good Education to all the Poor Children in England, at a moderate Expense* (Bath: R. Crutwell; London: Cadell and Davies, 1812).

30 in-scholars would be one-third of all the boys in Chester who were 9 years old, a figure that would include all those who needed charitable education for their children. At the same time, Haygarth was deeply concerned with the education of girls. He found that when his own parish started a school for girls, three-quarters of those aged between 9 and 13 could neither sew nor make a single article of dress. They were equally inept at knitting, an activity with which his grandfather had been involved as a hosier in his native dale and that in nearby Dent was a major source of income for the poor.

It was perhaps not surprising, given his strong Anglican connections, that Haygarth was deputed by his fellow trustees to approach the Lord Bishop of Chester, the Right Reverend Dr. Porteus, with a request that he preach a sermon in the cathedral in support of the measures then being adopted, at Haygarth's instigation, "to give a good education to the children of *all* our poor fellow citizens." Haygarth later told the Bishop, "I shall ever remember what heartfelt satisfaction I received from the benevolent remarks with which our petition was granted."[156] Porteus's sermon was duly printed in Chester but no copies appear to have survived.

Howard was clearly impressed by the steps taken in Chester for the education of the poor, so much so that he published, verbatim, *Report of the state of the Blue-Coat Hospital, in Chester, from the 1st of May 1786, to the 1st of May 1787*. He added, "To an ancient establishment of an *hospital* for *poor children*, a charity for the education of a large number of out-scholars has been annexed, and has been productive of the happiest results."[157] There were others who followed the Chester example. Dr. Briggs, a clergyman of Kendal, reorganized the Kendal Blue-Coat School so as to include a day school of industry for the children of the poor of his town.[158]

Lazarettos and the Plague

After John Howard's visit to Chester, he sent Haygarth his publication on lazarettos. There had been no epidemic of plague in England for over a hundred years. In 1720, London had been concerned about an outbreak of the disease in Marseilles and this led to Richard Mead publishing his *A Short Discourse concerning Pestilential Contagion and the Methods to be used to*

---

[157] Howard, *An Account of the Principal Lazarettos*, 123.

[158] Probably Thomas Briggs, curate of Natland, near Kendal, who died January 4, 1816, at age 53. Information provided by Richard Hall, Cumbria Record Office, Kendal.

Prevent it.[159] Mercifully, for reasons not at the time apparent to London's citizens, there had been no recurrence of the disastrous outbreak that afflicted London in 1665. Haygarth himself therefore had no personal knowledge of plague. Knowing nothing of the importance of rats in the transmission of the disease, he was, quite naturally, convinced in his own mind that the plague "spread by the same laws, as many other distempers common in this part of Europe; namely the smallpox, measles, chincough, scarlet fever, &c," all of which, as he had learned from William Cullen, were contagious. Because, as he put it, "The propagation of infectious diseases has been an object of my particular attention for nearly a dozen years,"[160] he had no hesitation in putting forward recommendations governing lazarettos based on his notions of the transmission of infectious disease. As to regulations, he thought that they should be founded on cleanliness and separation.

As was to be his practice many times in future years, he used a letter, to John Howard in this case, as a means of setting out his views. The letter, a long one, was dated Chester, May 30, 1789.[160] Quite apart from his desire to prevent infection from coming into England, Haygarth was concerned that the measures he proposed would encourage trade with Turkey and the Levant. He thought that the present regulations for lazarettos were extremely erroneous. Some expensive and tedious restrictions were superfluous and others were omitted that he thought necessary. There were, in his opinion, two main considerations. First, were the contents of a ship coming from a potentially infectious port, which could be purified on the voyage home. Second, was the ship's cargo, which had to be dealt with in an English lazaretto.

It was clearly necessary that the crew and their belongings should be kept scrupulously clean, in the same way that "the justly celebrated Captain Cook" had preserved the health of his seamen on his voyages around the world. Provisions were not to be considered infectious, nor sails or cables. Records should be kept of any symptoms of the plague that might be reported by those on board. If these procedures were followed, there would be no need for crew and passengers to be detained in quarantine on their arrival in an English port. It was different, however, for those involved in unloading cargo that might carry

---

[159] Richard Mead, *A Short Discourse concerning Pestilential Contagion and the Methods to be used to Prevent it* (London: S. Buckley, 1720). See also Patrick Russell, *A Treatise of the Plague* (London: G.G.J. and J. Robinson, 1781).

[160] J. Aikin, *Appendix (to the Account of the Lazarettos); containing observations concerning foreign prisons and hospitals, collected by Mr Howard, in his concluding tour. Together with two letters to Mr Howard from John Haygarth* (London: J. Johnson, 1791), 22–29. John Aikin was John Howard's literary executor.

the disease. The articles requiring purification in England were cotton, cotton yarn, silk, mohair yarn, goat's wool, carpets, and so on. Drugs such as opium, scammony, gums, and the like, and fruit, such as figs, often part of the cargo of Turkish ships, were never themselves deemed infectious, but the coverings in which they were packed might be. Because they were firmly battened down in the hold of the ship during transit, there was no way they could infect the crew on board. It was also important that an exact manifest of the ship's cargo, attested at the port of embarkation, should be presented in England on arrival. In order to combat possible infection, all the cargo should then be landed, stored in a lazaretto, and exposed to air. The time required for exposure was not necessarily longer than a few hours or even days, and the tedious business of quarantining for as long as forty days would be superfluous.

The lazaretto should be so designed as to provide suitable living accommodations for the crew or porters involved in dealing with the cargo. There should also be ample space for exposing items of cargo to a free flow of air. As Haygarth had concluded from his studies of smallpox, he considered that any possible poison was only infectious to a very short distance, so that those involved with dealing with a potentially infectious cargo should simply keep to windward of it.

Because this letter was written just before John Howard was to depart on his last journey, on this occasion to Holland, Germany, Prussia, Livonia, and Russia, Haygarth could not forbear from posing a number of questions in the manner that was his wont. He suggested that Howard might be able to collect some valuable facts, particularly because the plague had been devastating in cities such as Moscow and Kiev as recently as 1770. He wanted to know how the infection was communicated, at what time, and at what distance from an infected person, and how and when different members of the same family were attacked.

As to projected lazarettos in England, Haygarth thought that in addition to London and Bristol there should be such an institution in Liverpool, particularly because this would facilitate the importation of cotton from Turkey for the Lancashire and Cheshire manufacturers. He thought that Hilbree Island, situated at the confluence of the rivers Dee and Mersey, would be the most suitable location.

Haygarth was concerned that this letter would not reach Howard before his departure, and on being reassured that he had received it, wrote again from Chester, on June 19, 1789.[161] He told Howard that he was not at all

---

[161] Ibid, 30–32.

happy with his proposal to visit Barbary. He thought that so ignorant a people could not possibly afford him any useful information, nor, he wrote, were they "sufficiently intelligent to profit from his instruction." He concluded with his "sincerest good wishes for your help and happiness," but it may have been a premonition that led him to tell Howard that he sincerely regretted his journey, "so dangerous to a life of great importance to your country and mankind." His fears were to be realized by John Howard's death during that last journey. He contracted camp fever, presumably typhus, in Kherson, in South Russia, and died there on January 20, 1790.[162] Such was his fame that he was buried among a great concourse of people. As Edmund Burke had so cogently put it, in a much quoted phrase, he was ever ready "to dive into the depths of dungeons, to plunge into the infection of hospitals, to survey the mansions of sorrow and pain, to remember the forgotten, and to visit the forsaken."[163]

Nature, Cause, and Cure of the Rabies Canina

Working in a city with an extensive surrounding countryside where dogs were a necessary part of country life, Haygarth must have constantly seen patients suffering from rabies. It is therefore not surprising that in the same year that John Howard paid his visit to Chester he should comment on the treatment of this often fatal condition. On November 17, 1788, he wrote to Percival in Manchester setting out his proposal for dealing with the bite of a mad dog.[164] In that month there had been widespread alarm when three men of Wrexham, North Wales, died of "canine madness." Haygarth thought there was "a safe, easy and effectual method of preventing infection." It was well known that it was the spittle of the mad animal that caused the disorder, so the first thing to do was obviously to remove it with a dry cloth and then to wash the wound with cold water. This, he thought, should be continued in bad cases for several hours. Then warm water should be plentifully used, and "a continued stream of it, poured from the spout of a tea-pot or tea-kettle, held up at a considerable distance, is peculiarly well adapted to the purpose." Persistent washing in this way would clearly reduce the amount of

[162] John Howard, *An Account of the Principal Lazarettos in Europe: with various papers relating to the Plague: together with further Observations on some Foreign Prisons and Hospitals* (Warrington: W. Eyres and London: T. Cadell, 1789), 208–209.

[163] See Edmund Burke, *Works* (London: Hansard and Sons, 1815), vol. 3, 380–381.

[164] Thomas Percival, *Hints towards the investigation of the nature, cause, and cure of the Rabies Canina: Addressed to Dr Haygarth* (Manchester, 1789).

poison in the wound by progressive dilution. Later it might be necessary for a surgeon to excise the wound, particularly if it was deep. In any uncertainty he should cup and syringe. Haygarth asked that this paper should be put up in public places and "in the houses of several sensible and humane persons in each parish."

Percival responded by publishing Haygarth's letter as a pamphlet in Manchester. He began with an extensive review of what was known of rabies, citing Morgagni and other learned authors as well as particular case reports. He went on to conclude that Haygarth's suggestions were in the main judicious, though it might be necessary to place ligatures above and below the wound. He emphasized the uncertainty of the time that might elapse from the bite of the afflicted animal to the development of the classical symptoms of rabies. Various remedies were recommended, even the newly discovered foxglove, which might be expected to affect the brain powerfully, excite sickness and vomiting, and produce a copious flow of saliva. But at the end of the day he did not regard Haygarth's regimen as anything more than a rational hypothesis. He concluded with the hope that his hints might incite his friend to extend his researches. There were others in Manchester at that time whose interests were directed to the problem of rabies. Samuel Bardsley (1764–1851) published his observations on the "canine and spontaneous hydrophobia" in *Proceedings of the Manchester Literary and Philosophical Society* in 1793.[165]

The rabies paper does more than show the extent of Haygarth's constant interest in the problems of the day and the way in which he so frequently sought Percival's advice. It also provides evidence that he was still in touch with his old student friend, Arthur Lee of Virginia. After Edinburgh, Lee had been in London for a while before he returned to Virginia, where he briefly practiced medicine. He was soon back in London, where he now decided to study law; he was called to the bar in 1773. He became heavily involved in the politics of American independence, accompanying Benjamin Franklin, now effectively America's ambassador in France, to Paris after war broke out in 1775. After disagreements with Franklin, he settled in his native America in 1780, taking part in the political events that led to the foundation of that great new Republic. He was back in Virginia when his old friend, John Haygarth, sent him his description of his method for treating the bite

---

[165] S. A. Bardsley, "Miscellaneous observation on canine and spontaneous hydrophobia: to which is prefaced the history of a case of hydrophobia occuring twelve years after the bite of a supposed mad dog," *Memoirs of the Manchester Literary and Philosophical Society* 4 (1793): 431–488. See also Samuel Argent Bardsley (1764–1851), physician to Manchester Infirmary 1790–1823, *Oxford DNB;* 3:795.

of a mad dog. Lee sent it to the newspapers with his own endorsement. Writing from Philadelphia, John Morgan added a recommendation of his own. Lee died a few short years later, on December 12, 1792, at his home. He had called it Lansdowne after the English aristocrat, then Lord Shelburne, a close friend to America, whom he had known so well in his London days. It was the first death among John Haygarth's friends from his student days in Edinburgh.[166]

He was to lose others who had been loyal and close supporters of his work in Chester. His devoted friend, Thomas Falconer, had died in Chester on September 4, 1792. Bishop Porteus, another influential supporter in the city, had already left Chester. He had been translated to the bishopric of London in 1787.

An Annuity for a Poor Widow

John Haygarth was undoubtedly busy in 1789. Nevertheless, domestic matters always demanded his attention. Among his many other avocations, he found time to involve himself in the provision of an annuity for a Mrs. Bowers, who may well have been one of his servants. It was an era when life insurance was being increasingly developed by commercial interests in the city of London. Charles Potts, Haygarth's Chester lawyer, was instructed to explore with the Equitable Assurance Company in London the possibility of providing for "the poor widow." William Morgan replied on May 16, setting out the sort of arrangement that would be necessary in providing for the lady, then 52 years old and not in perfect health. Potts consulted Haygarth who, his mathematical bent to the fore, seems to have taken a close interest in how the annuity could be funded. Among the Haygarth papers at the Chester Record Office are several pages of detailed financial calculations in Haygarth's characteristic hand. Potts replied to Morgan on May 24, 1789, with proposals that he and Haygarth thought might be appropriate. Morgan wrote again on June 18 and August 14, emphasizing that the sums envisaged by Haygarth were not satisfactory and coming up with further detailed proposals and with a request for a declaration respecting "Mrs B's age." By the end of August, Haygarth had had enough. He wrote to Potts telling him that he had by now "spoke to Mrs Bowers, and at last obtained her final answer to approve the purchasing the annuity from the Equitable Assurance

---

[166] Bell, "Arthur Lee."

Society." He asked Potts to excuse "all this unprofitable trouble." In fact, he had already signed the agreement with the Society for Equitable Assurances on Lives and Survivorships. On August 22 the society acknowledged receipt from Dr. Haygarth of the sum of 54 pounds 16 shillings, this being the premium required for "the assurance of the sum of eighteen pounds annuity during the natural life of Mrs Susannah Bowers after the expiration of fourteen years." How long the lady survived to benefit from these arrangements is not known.[167]

---

[167] The papers relating to Mrs. Bowers's annuity are preserved in the Cheshire Record Office.

7

A Plan to Exterminate Smallpox in Great Britain

A National Scheme

*E*ver since the publication of his *An Inquiry How to Prevent the Smallpox* in 1784, John Haygarth had sought to ensure that his ideas would be brought to the attention of his contemporaries, not only in Great Britain but also in America. After it was published, a copy of the *Inquiry* had been sent to Benjamin Franklin, through the good offices of Dr. Percival. Franklin himself had a personal interest in inoculation against smallpox. He lost his 4-year-old son, Francis Folger, "the delight of all that knew him," to the disease in 1736 and he never forgot his grief. In 1759, during his first stay in England, he had persuaded William Heberden to publish *Some Account of the success of Inoculation for the Smallpox in England and America, together with plain Instructions by which any Person may be Enabled to perform the Operation and Conduct the patient through the Distemper.*[168] In 1788, Haygarth wrote to Franklin with a set of papers on the smallpox, now preserved in the Franklin Papers at the American Philosophical Society in Philadelphia, asking Franklin to "communicate them to his countrymen in whatever manner

---

[168] Haygarth's letter to Franklin, preserved among the Franklin Papers at the American Philosophical Society, Philadelphia, read, "Chester 15 December 1788. Dr Haygarth sends the enclosed paper to Dr Franklin, and, if he approves the opinions they inculcate, requests therefore he will communicate them to his countrymen in whatever manner he judges most likely to promote their success. A few years ago an *Inquiry how to prevent the Smallpox* was transmitted to Dr F from Dr H by their friend Dr Percival, which was sent as a token of respect in the Author, for his philosophical discernment and knowledge." A copy of Haygarth's *Inquiry* is in the Library of the Historical Society of Pennsylvania. Weaver, "John Haygarth," 165.

he judges most likely to promote their success." Haygarth was particularly concerned to know whether his views on prevention, and in particular the "Rules for Prevention" he had promulgated, were generally acceptable. He was at that time on the verge of initiating a nationwide consultation in England on the validity of his rules.

In 1787, he indicated his intentions in a letter to William Cullen in Edinburgh. Writing from Chester on January 10, 1787, he told Cullen how honored he had been with his remarks on the *Inquiry*.[169] He went on,

> I feel, and shall for ever acknowledge, the sincerest and most affectionate gratitude for such a favour. I am conscious of how much I owe, on this occasion, to your friendship. Your criticism contributed, in a very important manner, to diminish the imperfections of my little book, but shall, as you desired, be ever held sacred and private. I hope that you duly received a copy of the *Inquiry*, of which I requested your acceptance, as soon as it was printed.

What Haygarth really wanted, however, was Cullen's approval for what he was now proposing. He also would have liked to publish a letter from Cullen that would strengthen his contentions and give respectability to his publication. He wrote,

> As I have no doubt that you long ago made up your mind on this subject, I hope that it will not much intrude upon your time, and the constant concerns which constantly employ your attention, to favour me with an answer to one of the queries which I had proposed, now altered into the following, or any other form you please. "Q. 2d. Do the *Rules of Prevention* (p. 118) appear fully sufficient to prevent the Small Pox, as far as you can judge from facts which have fallen under your own observation, or which you have received on the evidence of credible testimony, either as stated in the *Inquiry* or by others?" Your former criticism, I solicited for my own private satisfaction. I now request the authority of your name, if you continue to think that this dreadful pestilence may be avoided by practical regulations, and if you judge that the propagation of such an opinion may be of service to mankind. We know one another too well to suppose that, on this or any other occasion, I have a wish that you should assist one word beyond full conviction. Though your entire approbation would give me great satisfaction, yet I should esteem, as much more important, the detection of doubtful facts, or false conclusions. To explain in what circumstances the *Rules of Prevention* are defective, would be of the greatest service to the cause, and give me the highest satisfaction.

[169] Thomson, *Life of William Cullen*, 640.

He went on to explain to Cullen how he had attempted to get general approval for his proposals, emphasizing how much he valued the opinions of those he consulted. But he particularly wanted Cullen's approbation:

> I send a circular letter, on this occasion, to my medical friends who honoured the MS. *Inquiry* with their remarks. You will think this an unusual, and perhaps an unwarrantable, method of establishing medical opinions; but to me the cause appears important, and to justify such a measure. I need not intimate the high authority of your name, and the wonderful influence it would have, not only in this island, but in every other part of the world enlightened by literature. I hope and believe that a spirit of benevolence and philanthropy would promote societies to prevent the natural Small Pox, if the means were generally allowed to be practicable. If such institutions were successful, the best foundation would be laid for a general law.

Haygarth concluded, somewhat peremptorily, "A short answer, either public or private, as soon as may be convenient" would be the highest obligation to him.

Cullen does not seem to have agreed to Haygarth's request to use his name. The letter is significant, however, in showing how during the next few years Haygarth was to solicit support for his ideas on the prevention of smallpox from as many of his medical friends as he was able to persuade to join his campaign. No reply to Haygarth's appeal for support from Cullen has been preserved, nor in his future publications does Haygarth mention his consultation with his former professor. Perhaps by then Cullen, whose mind became clouded in his last years, was no longer able to respond. He was to resign his chair in Edinburgh at the end of 1789, and he died two months later.

The results of Haygarth's consultations were published, together with his proposals to eradicate smallpox from Great Britain, in 1793. The work had a long and utopian title: *A Sketch of a Plan to exterminate the casual Small-Pox from Great Britain; and to promote general Inoculation; to which is added a Correspondence on the nature of Variolous Contagion with Mr Dawson, Dr Aikin, Professor Irvine, Dr Percival, Professor Wall, Professor Waterhouse, Mr Henry, Dr Clark, Dr Odier, Dr James Currie and on the best Means of preventing the Small-pox, and promoting inoculation, at Geneva; with the Magistrates of the Republic.*[170]

[170] John Haygarth, *A Sketch of a Plan to exterminate the casual Small-Pox from Great Britain; and to promote general Inoculation; to which is added a Correspondence on the nature of Variolous Contagion with Mr Dawson, Dr Aikin, Professor Irvine, Dr Percival, Professor Wall, Professor Waterhouse, Mr Henry, Dr Clark, Dr Odier, Dr James Currie and on the best Means of preventing the Small-pox, and promoting inoculation, at Geneva; with the Magistrates of the Republic*, 2 vols. (London: J. Johnson, 1793), vol. 2, 193–195.

The book was as long-winded as the title. There were two volumes and 570 pages. It began with an adulatory four-page dedication to the king, George III. Haygarth had no hesitation in employing the most fulsome prose he could muster:

> History hath recorded many illustratious actions by your MAJESTY'S ances-tors, during a long succession of ages. Among them all, the most truly glorious, and in all its probable consequences, the most beneficial to mankind, was the introduction of inoculation into Europe in the year 1721.

Haygarth clearly had a highly focused interpretation of history. Always dedicated to his cause, inoculation was clearly of more importance to him than either Agincourt or the Glorious Revolution of 1688. He went on,

> As your MAJESTY has graciously condescended to patronise the following proposal, it will, on that account, derive a superior claim to the attentive con-sideration of all men of knowledge, patriotism and humanity.

In his preface Haygarth pointed out at once that the present work was to be regarded as a sequel to the *Inquiry*. It was clear, however, that he was now very much more ambitious. He was seeking to extend the proposals outlined in the *Inquiry* from the purely local interests of the city of Chester to establish a national organization for the prevention of smallpox that would encompass the whole country.

He pointed out in his introduction that what he proposed was not entirely new. He had, he wrote, put forward his ideas on how to exterminate small-pox from Great Britain to Fothergill at Lea Hall as long ago as the summer of 1778. There had been several conferences between the two men. It had been on these occasions that Haygarth had met Waterhouse and learned of the measures taken in Rhode Island to prevent the spread of smallpox. On Fothergill's return to London that autumn, he had consulted a number of his medical friends about Haygarth's proposals. He wrote to his Chester friend, "I have mentioned thy intention of freeing this country from small-pox to divers of the faculty, and shall continue to do so, as it falls in my way. The proposal is received variously, but in exact proportion to their humanity." In another letter he went on, "I do not forget the business of the small-pox. I mention thy views and wishes as opportunity offers; and shall very cheerfully unite in doing everything in my power to promote an institution, which has as its object the banishment of so great a plague."[170]

Fothergill died in December 1780, and Haygarth recorded in the introduction to his *Sketch* his sorrow at losing so able and zealous an advocate. He went on to outline his views on transmission, repeating his view that it was contagion that was the effective mode of transmission not only of smallpox, measles, and scarlet fever but also, as he had stated to John Howard, of plague. He repeated his rejection of the theories of the importance of atmospheric miasmata of Sydenham's followers, who still claimed that epidemic disease was due to an unfavorable constitution of the air. He thought that some of the individuals who could most usefully help in setting up an organization for the prevention of smallpox were clergymen. He was particularly interested in the work of the "Rev Mr Stuart," grandson of Lady Wortley Montagu, who had been highly successful in promoting inoculation in his own parish of Luton in Bedfordshire.[171] William Stuart (1755–1822) was the son of the third Earl of Bute, who had married Mary, daughter of Lady Mary Wortley Montagu. He was vicar of Luton from 1779 until 1794. There, he encountered a severe outbreak of malignant smallpox that caused great terror throughout his parish. Stuart offered to have everyone inoculated at his own expense. Nearly 2,000 came forward and the inoculations were carried out with only the help of country nurses and a country practitioner.[172] Stuart was highly regarded as a clergyman; he later became bishop of St. Davids and went on to be archbishop of Armagh.

At the end of this part of his publication Haygarth set out his "Rules for Prevention," again posing the queries that had concluded the *Inquiry*. The most important part of his book, however, occupying pages 113 to 189, was his proposal for the institution of a public establishment. Haygarth proposed a hierarchy of three tiers of officials. There were to be 500 surgeon or apothecary inspectors who would, as in Chester, conduct inspections of houses throughout the kingdom. There would be 500 districts throughout the land, one for each inspector. Then there would be fifty physicians, one for each ten inspectors, who would supervise their work. Either the king or the Royal College of Physicians would in his opinion be appropriate to appoint these men. There would also be a supervising commission, five physicians

---

[171] J. A. Venn, *Alumni Cantabrigiensis,* part II (Cambridge: Cambridge University Press, 1954), vol. 6: 74. James Boswell introduced Stuart to Dr. Johnson in 1783 as a "gentleman truly worthy of being known to Johnson; being, with all the advantages of high birth, learning, travel and elegant manners, an exemplary parish priest in every respect." James Boswell, *The Life of Samuel Johnson, Ll D* (London: Macmillan, 1900), vol. 3, 278.

[172] Lady Louisa Stuart, *The Letters and Works of Lady Mary Wortley Montagu, with Introductory Notes,* Lord Wharncliffe, ed. (London: C. Bohn, 1861).

in London and three in Edinburgh, similarly appointed. There were to be general inoculations. The "Public Establishment" should be enacted by law and give rewards for information about outbreaks of smallpox, and would also ensure the proper observance of the "Rules of Prevention." Conversely, transgression was to be punished by a fine and if unable to pay the offender was to be publicly exposed in the nearest market town with a label on his breast saying, "Behold a villain who has wilfully and wickedly spread the small-pox." Haygarth recognized that his plan might be dismissed as too visionary, and that it might seem either "an extravagent and dangerous inovation" or an "invasion of personal liberty." He stressed that he was anxious to encourage a dispassionate and considered debate of his proposals and earnestly entreated his readers not to dismiss his ideas out of hand. He also included the calculations made for him by John Dawson of Sedbergh, whose advice he greatly valued, on the population increase that might be expected to occur were smallpox to be eradicated. He wrote, "I requested the favour of my mathematical friend, MR DAWSON, to compute what would be the increase in population in Great Britain, at different future periods, if the smallpox could be exterminated, estimating the rate of mortality in this and other diseases according to the register kept at Chester for six years, 1772, 3, 4, 5, 6, and 7. I subjoin his calculation." Dawson's results were as follows:[173]

Increase of inhabitants if

Period of years	30,000 survive annually	35,000 survive annually
10	281,932	328,909
20	527,694	615,643
30	737,322	860,209
40	910,800	1,062,600
50	1,048,146	1,222,837
60	1,149,342	1,340,899

Correspondence with Professional Colleagues

By far the largest part of Haygarth's *Sketch*, however, was devoted to his correspondence with many friends, asking particularly whether his "Rules for Prevention" were entirely correct and appropriate. The last 150 pages of the first volume and the entire second volume contain this material. In

[173] Haygarth. *Sketch of a Plan*, 143–145.

general most agreed with his plan, but there were many points of detail that they disputed. Several letters passed between Haygarth and John Aikin (1747–1822),[174] the Unitarian radical, now in Great Yarmouth. He was not entirely convinced by Haygarth's view on the solution of the variolous poison. William Irvine (1743–1787),[175] however, professor of clinical chemistry in the University of Glasgow, found the facts adduced by Haygarth to be well established. He thought the arguments convincing and the conclusions "fairly given." Thomas Percival, as might be expected, was entirely supportive, as was Professor Martin Wall (1747–1824),[176] writing as Lichfield Professor of Clinical Medicine at the University of Oxford. Thomas Henry (1734–1816),[177] a chemist and surgeon apothecary in Manchester who was a fellow of the Royal Society, was also "satisfied that your conclusions were just." John Clark of Newcastle[178] also agreed with most of the data presented. James Currie, writing from Liverpool, was particularly well qualified to comment on the use of general inoculation and isolation in the control of smallpox on slave ships, which he had found to be eminently successful. But he also pointed out perceptively that Haygarth's plan, to be effective, would require the interposition of government.

There was a long letter from De Gouttes, the secretary to the Syndick and Council of Health of Geneva. They had already received a copy of Haygarth's *Enquiry*, translated by "notre compatriote Monsieur le Docteur De la Roche." De Gouttes gave Haygarth a detailed account of how the problem of smallpox had been approached in Geneva. He told Haygarth that there were 35,000 inhabitants of the Republic of Geneva, of whom 26,000 lived in the city. There were, however, a large number of "strangers." Inoculation had begun in 1751 and there had been considerable success in preventing the disease among children. But he pointed out that in a country with a republican constitution it was not possible to coerce people, the liberty of the individual being a fundamental right, a view that coincided with James Currie's reservations. He concluded with questions for Haygarth on whether the smallpox society was still active, what it had cost, and what other

---

[174] John Aikin (1747–1822), *Oxford DNB;* 1:485–486.

[175] William Irvine (1743–1787), *Oxford DNB;* 29:372–373.

[176] Martin Wall (1747–1824), *Oxford DNB;* 56:915. Edward Gibbon remembered him as a "learned, ingenious and pleasant gentleman."

[177] Thomas Henry (1734–1816), *Oxford DNB;* 26:594–595.

[178] John Clark (1744–1805), *Oxford DNB;* 11:813–814. Founder of the Newcastle Dispensary and physician to the infirmary.

towns in England had adopted the Chester model. Haygarth responded that the society was no longer in operation but that other towns, such as Leeds, Liverpool, and Newcastle, had been successful in introducing general inoculation, particularly among the "opulant." He himself had been approached by the Royal College of Physicians of Edinburgh on ways of providing inoculation gratis to poor citizens, and towns such as Dumfries had followed his lead. Nowhere except Chester, however, had "any regulations been attempted to exclude the casual smallpox."

Odier in Geneva also replied in a letter communicated by De la Roche in Paris on his behalf. Daniel De la Roche was a talented translator who, as already noted, had published a French translation of Haygarth's *Inquiry*. Originally from Geneva, where he had been a member of the "Conseil de Deux-Cents" and one of those who prepared the *Pharmacopoeia Genevensis*, he settled in Paris after 1782 and became physician to the Hopital Necker.[179] He was "Medicin de Monseigneur le Duc d'Orleans, et du Regiment des Gardes Suisses, membre du College de Medecins de Geneve, et de la Societe Royale de Medicine d'Edinbourg." Odier wrote, "Il n'y a rien de plus difficile que de faire des observations precises sur la maniere dont se propagent les maladies contagieuses," and went on to attempt answers to Haygarth's queries. He did not think the "Rules of Prevention" were unnecessarily restrictive. He doubted, however, if every necessary restriction had been identified. As to the question of whether he had seen three or more persons afflicted, he thought possibly he had. He had no answer to Query 4 and thought that he had seen instances of transmission occurring through clothes and the like "every day." Louis Odier[180] was the first of a group of Geneva contemporaries who studied medicine in Edinburgh. He graduated MD in 1770 with a thesis entitled *De Musicae Sensationibus*. He also visited London.

The longest correspondence was between Haygarth and his old friend Benjamin Waterhouse in Boston, now the first professor of medicine at Harvard. There were four long letters from Boston with two detailed replies from Chester. The main bone of contention was whether smallpox could be

---

[179] Daniel De la Roche (b. 1743), *Dictionnaire Historique et Biographique de la Suisse* (Neuchatel: Administration du Dictionnaire Historique et Biographique de la Suisse, Vol. 2, 1924), 648–649.

[180] On Louis Odier (1748–1817), see Christopher Lawrence and Fiona A. Macdonald, eds., *Sambrook Court: The Letters of J. C. Lettsom at the Medical Society of London* (London: Wellcome Trust Centre for the History of Medicine at University College, 2003), 225. See also *Dictionnaire Historique et Biographique de la Suisse*, vol. 5, 1930; 180.

transmitted by the air across significant distances. Waterhouse believed that on one occasion it had passed from a patient in Boston to workmen across the Charles River. This was so contrary to Haygarth's essential thesis that it took considerable effort and much time before Waterhouse could be brought to accept that transmission could only take place over a very short distance.

One of the most succinct accounts of the success of Haygarth's "Rules of Prevention" was provided for him by his old friend, John Dawson of Sedbergh. Dawson described his experience of a single patient:

> A young man (John Airey) came from a distance with a fever upon him. It proved to be the smallpox and of the confluent kind; of which he died on the 28th or 29th day. He lodged in Finkle Street, which cannot be more than three yards broad. He lay up one flight of stairs; but at the head of them, where there was no door. The foot of the stairs is close to the door, which opens onto the street. The house where he was, being exceedingly small, and he a very lusty young man, there was not a particle of air but what was impregnated with the contagion, as might be discovered by the smell. Upon going into the house, the offensive stench struck one immediately; and as the door is a back one, I am pretty confident might have been perceived, before it was opened.
>
> No particular precaution was used by the uninfected, except by keeping out of the house. The nurses were desired to wash the dirty clothes, and to convey away all discharges &c from the patient, at proper hours.
>
> The smallpox has not been epidemical at Sedbergh for upwards of seven years. Some of the neighbours had not had the distemper, nor great amounts of children, who passed through the streets each day; yet not one caught the Infection.[179]

Haygarth clearly paid a great deal of attention to what his correspondents wrote, publishing their letters verbatim. It was his way of ensuring that his views were endorsed by his colleagues. He was therefore able justifiably to conclude with the statement that every conceivable doubt had been "scrupulously subjected to the public consideration."[170, 181]

The Public Response

It is all the more surprising, therefore, that Haygarth's *Sketch* had so little impact, in particular receiving no attention from those in authority. The *Gentleman's Magazine* did not even attempt to review it. His work was clearly

[181] Haygarth, *Sketch of a Plan,* 193–195.

to be eclipsed five years later by Jenner's demonstration of the value of vaccination. Yet Lobo has argued that there may have been political reasons.[182] The central political facts of the 1790s, he has argued, were entirely determined by the cataclysm of the French Revolution and the ambitions of revolutionary France. In the year that Haygarth's *Sketch* was published, France had declared war on England. English dissenters, many of whom had been supporters of American independence, were enthusiastic during that period about the events unfolding across the channel. Their unpopularity, however, was reflected in the Birmingham riots of 1791, when William Withering very nearly lost his house to rioters and when Priestley's home, his laboratory, and the records of his experiments were unceremoniously torched by the mob. It was also clear that several of Haygarth's correspondents, for example, James Currie, were known to be dangerous radicals. Currie, in addition to being a vehement opponent of slavery, was a notorious pamphleteer whose incendiary writings under the pseudonym "Jasper Wilson" had brought him into direct conflict with the national authorities. John Aikin had been forced to leave Great Yarmouth in 1792 because of his Unitarianism and his sympathy with the aims of the French revolutionaries. Even though Haygarth had praised the king in his fulsome dedication, Haygarth's dissenting associates were, as Lobo has pointed out, "immediately dismissable."

There were, however, other reasons why the book was not at once given its due. There had clearly been delays in distributing the book, possibly by the printer. Thomas Percival wrote from Manchester,

> The publication of your "Sketch..." I have not yet seen announced in the papers. * * * is a very honest man but he will stand in need of an occasional spur to his exertions. The delay in the conveyance of your work was mortifying; and I lament that the public is now so fully and solicitously engaged in the great political events of Europe, as to be less likely to pay due regard to your important proposals. However, you will have executed the office of a wise and patriotic citizen.[183]

But there was also another more prosaic explanation for its lack of success. Haygarth was invariably at his best when he wrote succinctly and with brevity. It has to be admitted that the *Sketch* is a tedious read. There must have been those whose hearts fell when the book thudded onto their desks in the summer of 1793. Significantly, perhaps, many of the pages in the

---

[182] Lobo, "John Haygarth."

[183] Percival, *Memoirs,* clxxiv.

second volume preserved in the library of the Royal College of Physicians in London remained uncut for more than 200 years. Perhaps Haygarth would have been better advised if he had simply published the section that included the details of his utopian plan and ensured its circulation among those who might have been able to promote it both locally and in Parliament.

For Thomas Percival, 1793 was particularly grievous. His second son, James Percival, a young man of great promise then finishing his medical studies in Edinburgh, died from a fever contracted from a patient. Haygarth's message of condolence, "a kind and consolatory letter," was received with grateful acknowledgment.[184] It was an event that saddened many. Anthony Fothergill had been a fellow student in Edinburgh with Thomas Percival. Writing from Bath to his protégé James Woodforde in Edinburgh, fellow student with James Percival, he told him how much he regretted "young Percival's death, the son of my venerable correspondent and contemporary, Dr. Percival."[185]

---

[184] Ibid., clxxvii.

[185] Christopher Lawrence, Paul Lucier, and Christopher C. Booth, *Take Time by the Forelock: The Letters of Anthony Fothergill to James Woodforde 1789–1813* (London: Wellcome Institute for the History of Medicine, 1997), 44.

From Chester to Bath

Last Years in Chester

*J*ohn Haygarth's *Sketch* was the last of his works to be published during his Chester years. His correspondence with Waterhouse continued. There had been queries from across the Atlantic about the way in which Haygarth's university, Cambridge, awarded its degrees. Perhaps as a reward for the information that he sent, Haygarth heard late in 1794 that he had been honored with both the MB and MD degrees. He could now, for the first time, use the initials MD after his name.

It was in that same year that Haygarth first heard that something was afoot in rural Gloucestershire. Edward Jenner's idea that cowpox could prevent smallpox was not then widely known, but on hearing of it Haygarth wrote at once to Jenner's ecclesiastical friend, Dr. Worthington, "I hope no reliance will be placed on vulgar stories, the author should admit nothing but what has been proved by his own personal observation, both in the brute and human species."[186] Haygarth need have had no concern for the scientific credentials of the humble country surgeon who had been John Hunter's favorite pupil and who was already a fellow of the Royal Society. Two years later, in 1796, Jenner first demonstrated that the boy James Phipps, inoculated in the arm with cowpox obtained from the hand of a milkmaid, Sarah Nelmes, could not then receive smallpox by inoculation of material from a smallpox patient. Jenner sent his account to his friend Everard Home, John Hunter's brother-in-law, for submission to the Royal Society. Home thought the account curious, but perfectly reasonably was not satisfied with a single case only, nor with the apparent paradox, pointed out by Jenner, that an

[186] John Baron, *The Life of Edward Jenner M. D., LLD, F.R.S.* (London: Henry Colburn, 1838).

individual might have cowpox twice. He wrote to Sir Joseph Banks, then president of the Royal Society, on April 22, 1797:

> I read over Jenner's paper, and think the account of the Cowpox curious, but dare not venture to be satisfied with the evidence there addressed that it is a prevention of Smallpox, for the following reasons. The same person can have the Smallpox only once, but the Cowpox Dr Jenner has met with twice in the same person, this is a strong characteristic difference. The persons who were not susceptible of the Smallpox after having had the Cowpox were grown persons and were probably not susceptible of that disease, and the instances are much too few to admit of conclusions being drawn from them—if 20 or 30 were inoculated for the Cowpox and afterwards with the Smallpox without taking it, I might be led to change my opinion. At present however I want faith.[187]

The medical world had to wait two more years before Jenner published his epoch-making work after carrying out further successful experiments.

By now Haygarth's highly successful practice was consuming his time entirely, but at the same time he wanted the opportunity to write up the large amount of unpublished material he had amassed during his Chester years. He decided to retire. The large house he had built on the north side of Foregate Street was sold to a Chester worthy by the name of Madam Bold. The house has not been preserved, but the present Bold Square, just off Foregate Street, marks the site of John Haygarth's Chester home.

The Royal Crescent

Haygarth's decision to move to Bath in 1798 may well have been prompted by his continuing friendship with William Falconer. While Haygarth soldiered on in Chester, Falconer, following his removal to Bath in 1770, had built up a large practice. He had a well-deserved reputation as a physician with a scientific bent.[188] He had written extensively on the use of mineral waters, using statistical analysis to assess the efficacy of treatment. He had been elected a fellow of the Royal Society as early as 1773. He was also a corresponding member of the Medical Society of London, founded by Lettsom that same

---

[187] Banks Letters, Royal Botanic Gardens, Kew; 2:159. See also Derek Blaxby, "Edward Jenner's Unpublished Smallpox Inquiry and the Royal Society: Everard Home's Report to Sir Joseph Banks," *Medical History* 43 (1995): 108–110.

[188] William Falconer (1744–1824), *Oxford DNB;* 18:976–977.

year. After Fothergill's death in 1780, Lettsom had established a gold medal in his memory to be awarded for an essay on a subject chosen by the society. The first Fothergillian Gold Medal was awarded by the Medical Society in 1788 to William Falconer.[189] The title of the essay, which would have been sent to his old friend in Chester, was *The Influence of the Passions upon Disorders of the Body*, a subject that was to be of great interest to Haygarth during his first years in Bath.[190] It was a work that was to go through several editions. Falconer wrote on the effects of fear and other passions, such as the imagination. He was outspoken in his dismissal of Mesmer, whose concept of animal magnetism, supposedly related to a variety of disorders, was highly dubious. Falconer described how the commissioners charged by the French king with the examination of animal magnetism and chaired by Benjamin Franklin had proved "by the most decisive experiments, that the imagination alone is capable of producing all those convulsive effects, which have been falsely attributed to the power of the magnet." On the power of suggestion he quoted James Lind, who in his work on the prevention of scurvy wrote that he was always wary of fictitious cures, warning of the "wonderful and powerful influence of the passions of the mind upon the state and disorders of the body."

William Falconer lived in some style in the Circus in Bath. He did not always make a favorable impression upon those he met. In October 1794, Katherine Plymley, a lady from Shropshire visiting Bath, recorded in her diary,

> We dined at Dr Falconers in the family way. [He] is a man of great talents & great learning . . . an excellent physician & a good benevolent man, a good Husband & a good father, yet for want I will not say of courtesy only, but of common civility, he does not please. He walks about his house with so much rude inattention, not to say apparent contempt of his guests.[191]

Mrs. Falconer, however, was quite different. She showed the Shropshire visitor much kindness, which "took all my attention." She receives company, wrote Mrs. Plymley, every Monday evening. The house, she went on,

---

[189] Christopher C. Booth, "The Fothergillian Medals of the Medical Society of London," *Journal of the Royal College of Physicians London* 15 (1981): 254–258.

[190] William Falconer, *A Dissertation on the Influence of the Passions upon Disorders of the Body, being an Essay to which the Fothergillian Medal was adjudged* (London: C. Dilly and T. Phillips, 1788). This work went through four editions.

[191] Ellen Wilson, *A Shropshire Lady in Bath 1794–1807*, Bath History, vol. 4 (Bath: Millstream Books, 1992).

Is a handsome one in the Circus, dining parlour & library below, two drawing rooms above. These drawing rooms open into each other, one is appropriated to cards, the other to conversation & work. We went to her party yesterday. Form is excluded & the meeting is pleasant. . . . Tea & coffee of course. Cakes, wine, ozyot, lemonade, ice &c are several times handed about & the company all retire by 10 o'clock.[189]

It was to the nearby Royal Crescent that Haygarth moved. A letter written by him from "Bath Crescent" to Thomas Pennant, the distinguished naturalist and travel writer,[192] is dated June 18, 1798, suggesting that he moved into his Bath home during the summer of that year. Thomas Pennant, from Downing in Flintshire, the adjacent county to Cheshire, was a patient of Haygarth, who refers to him as his neighbor and gives advice on the measures he should adopt to counter his present ill health. Haygarth's advice seems to have been of little avail, for Pennant died in December of that year. Haygarth told Pennant of the help that the Falconers were giving to him and his family. Clearly Dr. Falconer was more at home with his close friends than with visitors whom he hardly knew. "Dr and Mrs Falconer," Haygarth wrote, "have been most friendly to us; they are our chief associates. I was at their house yesterday evening. . . . The Doctor had made frequent inquiries concerning your welfare." Haygarth also gave Pennant news of his own family. "All my invalids are much better since their departure from Chester. The journey was of service to each, & the Bath water to some." He reassured Pennant, "Wherever we may wander, our hearts will always be warmly attached to our old neighbours."[193] Haygarth subsequently bought No. 15, The Royal Crescent and lived there until 1812.[194]

Bath would be a very different environment from provincial Chester. The city had been known for its waters since Roman times, but it was during the eighteenth century that Bath became a center for the wealthy and fashionable, drawn to the city by its waters and by the opportunity of being seen in the company of the social elite of the land. It was in Bath that the upper

[192] Thomas Pennant (1726–1798), *Oxford DNB;* 15:765–768. John Haygarth had known Pennant since his first visit to Chester during his Welsh tour of 1773, when he noted Haygarth's finding that the proportion of deaths to the number of inhabitants in Chester was more favorable than in cities such as Leeds or London.

[193] Autograph letter, John Haygarth to Thomas Pennant, Bath Crescent, 18 June 1798, Warwickshire County Record Office, CR 2017/TP151/13.

[194] Dr. Haygarth's ownership of No. 15, The Royal Crescent, from 1800 until 1819, is recorded in the title deeds of the property. Personal communication, 14/8/1961, from T. H. Spencer Tizzard, then the owner of the property.

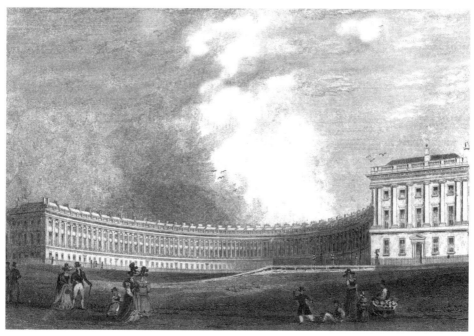

FIG. 5. The Royal Crescent Bath, early nineteenth century
(Courtesy of Frederika Cards Ltd, Bath.)

classes played cards, attended masked balls, took the waters, and laughed at the plays of Sheridan, while in the background the doctors, obsequious and guinea-collecting, hovered discreetly. The environment of Bath was anathema to the strict Quaker Fothergill, who, despite having recommended the city to William Falconer, thought it the "place that I should choose to reside in the last of all others. The people are accustomed to behave well to everybody while present, but more than that they don't seem to think is expected or necessary."[195] The more worldly Dr. Haygarth clearly found Bath congenial, as did his wife. He now retired completely from active practice and devoted himself to literary and philanthropic work, only responding occasionally to letters asking for advice.

When Haygarth arrived in Bath it was the city of Sheridan and Jane Austin.[196] The magnificent Royal Crescent, designed twenty years earlier by William Wood the Elder, was then, as now, the most prestigious address in

[195] Corner and Booth, *Chain of Friendship*, 94.

[196] R. A. L. Smith, *Bath* (London: B. T. Batsford, 1944).

town and the chosen resort of the elite. As Jane Austin put it in *Northanger Abbey*, it was to the Royal Crescent that the Allens and the Thorpes repaired "to breathe the fresh air of genteel company." It had been from the Royal Crescent that Sheridan had eloped with Miss Linley. The sybaritic Duke of York was one of Haygarth's neighbors.

Haygarth's wife Sarah seems to have emulated her neighbor Mrs. Falconer in the parties that she regularly organized. In January 1807, Katherine Plymley, whose comments on the Falconer household have already been noted, recorded,

> We went with Mrs Corbett to a large party at Mrs Haygarths. Dr Haygarths is an elegant house in the Crescent. The drawing room is large, four windows in front handsomely furnished. Another room backwards was opened. I was told above four hundred cards were sent out & it was supposed that in the course of the evening not many fewer persons were there. . . . Refreshments, tea, ice, oziyat &c handed out in abundance.[197]

In the world of Bath medicine, Haygarth found himself among eminent men. Falconer introduced him to the Bath Literary and Philosophical Society. The society, similar to other provincial societies of the time, was a successor to a society founded in 1777, originally to encourage "Agriculture, Planting, Manufactures, Commerce and the Fine Arts." Falconer was a founder member, as was Crutwell, later to be Haygarth's publisher in Bath. Priestley was a member of the society when he was living at Bowood, Lord Shelburne's home near Bath. Haygarth had good reason to write to his friend Thomas Percival, "On my change of situation, you will think me uncommonly fortunate in being placed at Bath so eminently distinguished for the liberality, charity, and superior knowledge of its inhabitants."[198]

For some years the Bath Philosophical Society was to meet weekly at Haygarth's house, an assembly of men of science for the purpose of mutual communication and free discussion of philosophical subjects. Apart from William Falconer, other distinguished inhabitants of the city included the friend and colleague to whom Jenner was to dedicate his work on vaccination, Caleb Hillier Parry, later to be remembered for his work on the effects of overactivity of the thyroid gland. Haygarth may have already known Parry, for he was educated at the dissenting Academy in

[197] Ellen Wilson, *A Shropshire Lady in Bath 1794–1807,* Bath History, vol. 4 (Bath: Millstream Books, 1992).

[198] Baron, *Life of Edward Jenner,* 640.

Warrington.[199] Anthony Fothergill (namesake but no relation to Dr. John) was practicing in Walcot Parade on the London Road. Born in Ravenstonedale, he had like Haygarth been educated at Sedbergh School and Edinburgh. He was an early supporter of the Royal Humane Society.[200] Curiously, there is no evidence that Haygarth ever met Edward Jenner, from nearby Berkeley, or that he visited Thomas Beddoes at his Pneumatic Institute at Hotwells in Bristol. There Humphry Davy was working on nitrous oxide, and he put paid to the extraordinary suggestion by S. L. Mitchill of New York that the gas was an agent of contagion. A matter of considerable interest to the contagionist John Haygarth, Davy simply showed that animals could be safely exposed to the gas without ill effect. Furthermore, he could breathe it himself without experiencing any "remarkable effects."[201] Others, however, responded differently. Davy's discovery excited much curiosity among his friends, particularly the poets Wordsworth, Southey, and Coleridge. They all recorded their feelings after breathing Davy's gas. Southey, in particular, was wildly enthusiastic. He wrote, "Such a gas has Davy discovered—the gaseous oxide. . . . Davy has invented a new pleasure for which language has no name. I am going for more this evening."[202]

The *Variolae Vaccinae*

Jenner's epoch-making publication of *An Inquiry into the Causes and Effects of Variolae Vaccinae*—literally, smallpox of the cow—aroused great interest when it came out in the year that Haygarth moved to Bath.[203] It was dedicated to his Bath friend, Caleb Hillier Parry. Parry knew Jenner well. In his *Syncope Anginosa*, to be published the following year, he quoted some of Jenner's work on the appearance of the heart at autopsy in cases of angina pectoris. He was also to play an important role in the breeding of the Merino

[199] Sholem Glaser, *The Spirit of Enquiry: Caleb Hillier Parry, M.D., F.R.S.* (Stroud:, Alan Sutton, 1995).

[200] Christopher C. Booth, "The Two Fothergills," in *A Physician Reflects* (London: Wellcome Centre for the History of Medicine, 2003).

[201] Sir Harold Hartley, *Humphry Davy* (London: Nelson, 1966).

[202] Humphry Davy, *Researches, Chemical and Philosophical: Chiefly Concerning Nitrous Oxide* (London: J. Johnson, 1800), 507–509.

[203] Edward Jenner, *An Inquiry into the Causes and Effects of the Variolae Vaccinae* (London: Sampson Low, 1798).

sheep that came to mean so much to the economy of the newly founded colony of New South Wales. Parry was an important supporter of Jenner, as was the surgeon Thomas Creaser, who early in 1799 proposed setting up a society or institution for vaccination of the people of Bath.[204] There were many skeptics who derided Jenner's discovery, particularly among cartoonists, who depicted people growing horns after vaccination, but there were others who immediately endorsed the practice. Lettsom in London sent a copy of Jenner's *Inquiry* to Waterhouse in Boston as soon as it appeared, and Waterhouse published the news of Jenner's discoveries in the Boston newspapers as early as 1799. Haygarth was a supporter of Jenner from the outset. He was involved in setting up the Vaccine Institution in Bath, the first to be established in England. Within a year Waterhouse in Boston had received vaccine from Haygarth, and he at once successfully vaccinated his son and six members of his household.[205] There were others in America who set out to try the new vaccine. John Chichester in Charleston, South Carolina, carried out a vaccination in 1799. In New York, David Hosack had received threads impregnated with vaccine from George Pearson in London, but two attempts at vaccination failed. There were others who attempted to use the new vaccine, but Waterhouse was the only one to persevere, becoming the pioneer of vaccination in America. He was criticized, however, for attempting to preserve the practice for himself. A vinegary character in later years, he was to be known as the Jenner of America. The story that in his old age, Oliver Wendell Holmes could recollect the experience of being vaccinated as a child, seated upon the knee of Dr. Waterhouse is probably apocryphal.

---

[204] Glaser, *The Spirit of Inquiry.*

[205] Haygarth's vaccine was obtained from Dr. Jenner's stock by Creaser. See John B. Blake, *Benjamin Waterhouse and the Introduction of Vaccination: A Reappraisal* (Philadelphia: University of Pennsylvania Press, 1957).

Medical Publications and Other Activities

Metallic Tractors and the Power of the Imagination

*A*lthough the vaccination story was the major event to excite the interest of Bath society in 1798, there was at the same time a craze that Haygarth and Falconer determined to expose as the fraud it so obviously was. Perkins's Metallic Tractors, a simple pair of metal rods no more than a few inches long, were all the rage in Bath.[206] They were the brainchild of an American physician, Dr. Elisha Perkins of Plainfield Connecticut.[207] It was an era when, as in Paris, dubious claims were being made to exploit the mysterious force that was electricity. In 1791 Galvani had published his observations showing that the contraction of the muscles of a frog could be due to the agency of electricity. There were serious scientists who interested themselves in what they termed "medical electricity," for example, Charles Hunnings Wilkinson of London and Bath.[208] In France, Mesmer had made great claims for the importance of animal magnetism, a concept totally rejected by

[206] W. J. Bishop, "Elisha Perkins and His Metallic Tractors," *British Journal of Rheumatism* 1 (1939): 193–206. This excellent article, by a distingushed librarian, is the best and most comprehensive account of the Metallic Tractors affair. See also Roger Rolls, *The Hospital of the Nation: The Story of Spa Medicine and the Mineral Water Hospital at Bath* (Bath: Bird Publications, 1988).

[207] H. T. Elisha Perkins, *Dictionary of American Biography,* (London: Humphrey Milford, Oxford: The University Press, New York: Charles Scribner's Sons, 1934) 114:466–467. See also John Vaughan, *Observations on Animal Electricity in Explanation of the Metallic Operator of Dr Perkins* (Wilmington, Delaware, 1797).

[208] J. L. Thornton, "Charles Hunnings Wilkinson," *Annals of Science* 23 (1967): 198–202.

Benjamin Franklin and his commissioners. Perkins always claimed that his Metallic Tractors depended for their action "on the Galvanic principle." In fact, as Haygarth and Falconer were to show, he was as great an impostor as Mesmer or James Graham, with his Temple of Hymen and his Celestial Bed. There were many others in London, for example, Drs. Myersbach and Brodum, who successfully hoodwinked the public for financial advantage.[209] The public was gullible, almost eager to be fleeced. As Hogarth's famous print shows, the visit to a quack doctor was a feature of eighteenth-century life.

Perkins was an unlikely quack, coming from an old New England family and the son of a conventional and highly respected doctor. According to his son's account, he first noted during the 1780s that metallic instruments might cause contraction of a muscle during a surgical operation and that pain might be relieved by the application of a metallic object.[210] By 1795 he had sufficiently convinced himself and invented his Metallic Tractors. They were in fact two rods of metal a few inches long—one half round and pointed at the end whereas the other was flat with the name "Perkins Patent Tractors" stamped upon it. Naturally, the composition of the Tractors was kept secret. They were to be applied to the affected part and it was sometimes necessary to rub hard enough to produce redness. His report to his fellow members of the Connecticut Medical Society was received with considerable skepticism, and he was to be expelled for peddling a patent nostrum. But he patented his tractors in Philadelphia, then the nation's capital, and, remarkably, obtained the support of some of the most distinguished people in the land, including President George Washington as well as the chief justice of the Supreme Court. Apparently believing in the efficacy of his tractors and other patent medicines, however, he came to grief in New York in 1799, succumbing to an attack of pestilential fever.

His son Benjamin, an undoubted rogue and impostor, had in the meantime traveled to England, where he took out a British patent. He settled at No. 28 Leicester Square, which had been John Hunter's house, a shrewdly calculated move. London, "the needy villain's general home" to use Johnson's telling phrase, was swept with enthusiasm for the Tractors, which promised so much.[211] Bath too, a veritable paradise for the quack, was to fall for the

[209] J. J. Abraham, *Lettsom: His Life, Times, Friends and Descendants* (London: Heinemann, 1933).

[210] Benjamin Perkins, *The Influence of Metallic Tractors on the Human Body &c.* (London: J. Johnson and Ogilvy and Son, 1798).

[211] See Roy Porter, *Health for Sale: Quacks in England 1660–1850* (Manchester: Manchester University Press, 1989).

Tractors. Benjamin Perkins had an agent there, the surgeon Charles Cunningham Langworthy, who promoted the Tractors in Bath on his behalf. He had moved from Bristol to establish what he called a "Metallic practise." Langworthy himself had published an account of the supposed benefits of the Metallic Tractors.[212]

It is not difficult to imagine what Falconer, with his known views on the effects of imagination on bodily disorders, would have thought of Perkins's Metallic Tractors. Haygarth, practical and pragmatic, would no doubt have been equally skeptical. The two friends now decided to devise an experiment that would put the Tractors to the test. What they agreed to do was set out in a letter written by Haygarth to Falconer: "The Tractors have obtained such high reputation at Bath, even among persons of rank and understanding, as to require the particular attention of physicians." He went on,

> Let their merit be impartially investigated. . . . Prepare a pair of false, exactly to resemble the true Tractors. Let the secret be kept inviolable, not only from the patient, but every other person. Let the efficacy of both be impartially tried, beginning always with the false Tractors. The cases should be accurately stated, and the reports of the effects produced by the true and false Tractors be fully stated, in the words of the patients.[213]

The false Tractors were in fact made of wood, a material that could clearly not be influenced by either electricity or any spurious animal magnetism.

The tests were carried out over two days at the Bath Infirmary, in the presence of Haygarth and Falconer, and by Richard Smith, surgeon in Bristol. Equal effects were obtained with both the true and the false Tractors. Furthermore, the same results could be obtained by using pieces of bone, slate pencils, and painted tobacco pipes. Haygarth at once presented his findings to the Bath Literary and Philosophical Society and he went on to publish them in 1800, in a pamphlet dedicated to Falconer "as a memorial of a mutual, cordial and constant friendship for

[212] Charles Cunningham Langworthy, *A View of Perkinian electricity, or, an enquiry into the infuence of metallic tractors founded on a newly-discovered principle in Nature, and employed as a remedy in many painful inflammatory disorders &c.* (Bath: R. Crutwell, 1798). Langworthy (1771–1847) obtained an MD from the University of St. Andrews and was the proprietor of Kingsdown House at Box near Bath. This was a private mental asylum. Personal communication, Dr. Roger Rolls of Bath.

[213] John Haygarth, *On the Imagination as a Cause and as a Cure of Disease of the Body exemplified by fictitious Tractors and Epidemical convulsions* (Bath: R. Crutwell, 1800).

thirty-six years." It was entitled *On the Imagination as a Cause and as a Cure of Disease of the Body exemplified by fictitious Tractors and Epidemical convulsions*.[213] Haygarth, like Falconer, already knew of examples of disorders being caused by the imagination, for he also described in this paper cases of hysterical convulsions seen during his practice in Chester that he considered entirely due to suggestion. He had delivered a blow, which if not immediately devastating, was to prove mortal to the reputation of Perkins's Metallic Tractors.

The results of his study spread rapidly among the practitioners of Bath. Anthony Fothergill wrote in November 1799 to a friend telling him that "Dr Haygarth on the Tractors is in the press."[214] Haygarth, however, was concerned to ensure that his findings be distributed much more widely. He wrote to Cadell and Davies, his publishers, in January 1800 telling them, "As the poison is widely dispersed, so shd be the antidote."[215] Sixty-three copies were to go to Bristol, fifty copies were to supply the demand in Bath, and further copies were to go to Dublin and Cork as well as different towns in England. He also listed more than fifty individual physicians and friends who were to receive copies. They included his old friend William Herberden, Sir Lucas Pepys, Robert Willan, and Lettsom in London, as well as others in Chester (Thackeray, for example), Manchester (Thomas Percival), Liverpool (James Currie), and Edinburgh (Monro, Duncan, and Gregory).

The pamphlet was widely reviewed, but it was the *Gentleman's Magazine* that was the most perceptive. The editor wrote,

> We seldom remember in the course of our medical criticisms to have received more pleasure or satisfaction than what the perusal of this short but excellent essay hath afforded us. From a subject so apparantly barren and useless as that of the metallic tractors, which, in point of medical as well as mechanical virtues, have always in our estimation ranked *much below* those of a tenpenny nail, we little expected to meet with a most useful and ingenious publication, entitled from its intrinsic merit, to the serious perusal and attention of every practitioner.[216]

Others repeated Haygarth's experiment. A farmer in the West Country gathered his fellow villagers on the green and after producing

[214] Lawrence, Lucier, and Booth, *"Take Time by the Forelock,"* 78.

[215] Autograph letter, John Haygarth to Cadell and Davies, Bath, January 1800, from the collection of the Wellcome Library for the History and Understanding of Medicine, London.

[216] *Gentleman's Magazine*, March 1800, 70:253.

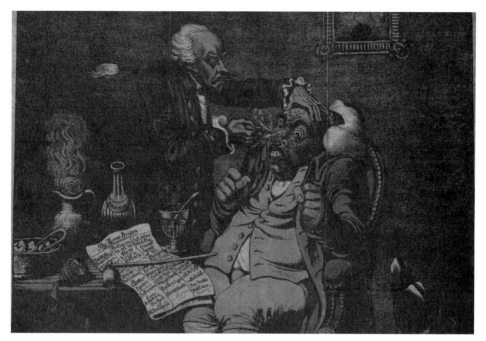

FIG. 6. Metallic Tractors, James Gillray, 1802
(Courtesy of the Wellcome Library, London.)

a burn on the paw of his dog, Pompey, showed them that the Tractors, which were supposed to be effective in veterinary practice, had no effect whatsoever. Pompey retired howling to his kennel.[217] The cartoonists soon joined the fray. Gillray's "Metallic Tractors," published in 1802, portrayed Benjamin Perkins attempting to treat a carbuncle on the alcoholic nose of John Bull with his Tractors. Charles Williams followed with a drawing of a society lady to whose venomous tongue the tractors were being applied. As Dr. Johnson put it, "Cheats can seldom stand long against laughter."[218]

Nevertheless, it took time for the fashion for the Tractors to die out. Society was then, as now, a slave to fashion. A correspondent wrote to the *Gentleman's Magazine*, "Are we not . . . governed by Fashion, and frequently

---

[217] John Corry, *The detection of Quackery; or, an analysis of medical, philosophical, political, dramatic, and literary imposture* (London: B. Crosby, 1802).

[218] Roy Porter, *Bodies Politic: Disease, Death and Doctors in Britain, 1650–1900* (London: Reaktion Books, 2001).

made a victim by it? And while we find five guineas for a pair of tractors, the poor perish for lack of food at our doors?"[219]

Benjamin Perkins continued in his publications to extol the virtues of his father's Tractors, quoting endlessly the cures wrought by them and letters from the influential people who supported him. He dismissed Haygarth as having "made a great noise" and having circulated his findings with remarkable industry in order to discredit the Metallic Tractors.[220]

By 1803 a Perkinian Institute had even been opened in Soho for the treatment of the poor. There was an imposing committee, with Lord Rivers as president and Governor Franklin, of all people, son of Benjamin Franklin who had so mercilessly exposed Mesmer in Paris, as one of the vice presidents. There was a grand opening dinner at the Crown and Anchor tavern on July 15, 1803. A poetical address was delivered, which began,

> See Pointed Metals, blest with power t'appease,
> The ruthless rage of merciless disease,
> Oer the frail part a subtil fluid pour,
> Drench'd with invisible Galvanic Shower,
> Till the arthritic, staff and crutch forego,
> And leap exulting like a bounding roe![219]

There were also still those who wrote in defense of the Tractors. In 1803, Thomas Green Fessenden, an American like Perkins, writing under the pseudonym of Sir Christopher Caustic MD, LLD, published a satirical poem addressed to the Royal College of Physicians that was supposedly an attack on Perkinism but was in reality a clever defense of the Tractors and a satire on orthodox medicine.[221]

In 1809, however, Lord Byron could write,

> What varied wonders tempt us as they pass!
> The cow-pox, tractors, galvanism and gas,

---

[219] Bishop, "Elisha Perkins and His Metallic Tractors."

[220] Benjamin Douglas Perkins, *The efficacy of Perkins Metallic Tractors on the human body and animals . . . to which is prefixed a preliminary discourse, in which, the fallacious attempts of Dr Haygarth to detract from the merits of the tractors, are detected and fully confuted* (London: J. Johnston, 1800).

[221] Christopher Caustic, MD, LLD (T. S. Fessenden), *A Poetic Petition against Tractorian Trumpery, and the Perkinian Institution, in four cantos . . . Addressed to the Royal College of Physicians* (London: T. Hurst and J. Ginger, 1802).

In turns appear, to make the vulgar stare,
Till the swoln bubble bursts—and all is air.

But before the bubble burst, Benjamin Perkins had escaped to his native America with, it was said, £10,000 profit in his pocket. Some might think it was only justice that he died in New York City in 1810 at the early age of 36.

In many ways, Haygarth's piece on the Metallic Tractors, which led him to set out his views on the importance of the imagination in medical conditions, was one of his best publications. He clearly showed that science is the only way to destroy a quack; denunciation is never enough, as Lettsom found to his cost when he tried unsuccessfully to unmask the infamous Dr. Brodum. Furthermore, Haygarth was one of the first to carry out a single blind clinical trial using a placebo.[222]

A New Century

A new century dawned. The long war with France was to stretch on, with only a brief respite following the Peace of Amiens in 1802, to Trafalgar and the battlefield of Waterloo. In 1801, to the consternation of his court and the alarm of his government, the king had a recurrence of the illness that had first afflicted him in 1788. But for the medical world of Bath it was the cowpox vaccination that occupied all minds. Anthony Fothergill wrote at the end of 1800 to his correspondent James Woodforde, "The cowpox continues to absorb the attention of the medl world beyond all other subjects."[223] Lettsom's new publication on vaccination was expected daily. Published in 1801, Lettsom's *Observations on the Cow-pock* provided important support from the capital for Edward Jenner. At the same time, Haygarth published a second edition of his *Inquiry* in which he presented himself as a zealous advocate of Jenner's vaccine inoculation.[224] Thomas Percival in Manchester, to whom Jenner had sent a copy of the *Variolae Vaccinae* as soon as it was

---

[222] Ulrich Trohler, *To Improve the Evidence of Medicine: The 18th Century British Origins of a Critical Approach* (Edinburgh: Royal College of Physicians of Edinburgh, 2000), 93. Roger Rolls, *The Hospital of the Nation: the story of spa medicine and the Mineral Water Hospital at Bath* (Bath: Avonlea Bird Publications, 1988).

[223] Lawrence, Lucier, and Booth, *"Take Time by the Forelock,"* 84.

[224] John Haygarth. *An Inquiry How to Prevent the Smallpox,* 2d ed. (Bath: R. Crutwell, 1801).

published, had urged Haygarth to engage in correspondence with Jenner, and it may have been Jenner himself who engaged Haygarth's enthusiastic interest. Haygarth now wrote,

> The discovery of Vaccine Inoculation by Dr Jenner is the most fortunate and beneficial improvement that medical science ever accomplished. It does not, however, preclude the necessity of investigating the variolous poison, and of considering by what regulations its propagation may be prevented. In order to secure the unthinking multitude from this destructive Pestilence, measures to prevent the casual Small-pox should everywhere accompany Vaccine inoculation. . . . I had the good fortune successfully to convey the first Vaccine Contagion to the inhabitants of America through Professor Waterhouse.[224]

It was also Haygarth who provided vaccine to Odier and his colleagues in Geneva. As he wrote in the second edition of his *Enquiry*, the new vaccine was "a discovery which can effectively destroy the Small-pox, the most mortal enemy that ever affected mankind." It was to be nearly 200 years before that utopian aim was achieved. The notion that smallpox could, as Haygarth had suggested, be effectively destroyed was not seriously considered until Victor Zdanov, vice minister of health in the Soviet Union, proposed to the World Health Assembly in 1958 that the global eradication of smallpox should be undertaken.[225]

The Control of Infectious Fevers

In the meantime, John Haygarth was addressing himself to his self-imposed task of putting together for publication the information that he had gathered during his Chester years. In 1800, he published a paper in the *Medical and Physical Journal* in London, "On Fever from Venereal Poison," reporting three cases of infection of the finger with "a low nervous fever," all occurring in surgeons or accoucheurs who had contracted venereal disease in the course of their work.[226] But the most important of the publications of those early years in Bath was his *Letter to Dr Percival on the Prevention of Infectious Fevers*.[227]

[225] F. Fenner, D. A. Henderson, L. Arita, and I. D. Lanyi, *Smallpox and Its Eradication* (Geneva: World Health Organization, 1988).

[226] John Haygarth, "On Fever from Venereal Poison," *Medical and Physical Journal* 3 (1800):198–203.

[227] Haygarth, *Letter to Dr Percival*.

Haygarth's work on establishing fever wards at the infirmary in Chester had at that time only been published in John Howard's works in 1792. His observations had been discussed by the group of physicians that met in Warrington and had formed part of his correspondence with colleagues such as Percival in Manchester and James Currie in Liverpool, as well as with physicians in Dublin and elsewhere. But it was now time to put this material on record. As with his other work in Bath, he first presented it to the Bath Literary and Philosophical Society, then published a hardback volume with Crutwell. The *Letter to Dr Percival* was a clear and comprehensive account of the fever wards at Chester and their success in preventing the spread of common infectious fevers. It was perhaps his best work. It was concise and clear, brief and succinct, and reads as freshly today as when it was written.

The *Letter* begins with an extensive section on preliminary principles. Haygarth describes how the Manchester physicians first established their board of health and how they went on to found their House of Recovery. He goes back to his first proposal for the establishment of fever wards in 1774, and later in 1783, emphasizing that houses that were "small, close, crowded and dirty" were particularly liable to harbor infectious fevers. As to the fever he was describing, he included "low, slow, nervous, putrid, petechial, malignant, pestilential, jail, ship, camp, hospital &c Fever, or Typhus." His first observations of the nature of febrile infection had been made in 1781, when he described the case of Mr. Cheers, who on April 21 of that year made a journey to Manchester, Cheadle, and elsewhere and was attacked by fever at his home on May 22, twenty-seven days after his return. Sixteen other members of his family were to be afflicted. Haygarth went on to describe the symptoms of the disease in some detail. He then set out the details of the cases of individuals he had observed, together with the reports of two apothecary surgeons, Mr. Connah and Mr. Manning. These were given in a series of tables. In Table I he described twenty different families, comprising 103 individuals, each identified by name, with the dates on which they were attacked by fever and how many days after exposure that was. There were detailed accounts of individual cases. Mrs. Deakin, for example, a charwoman, had been taken into the house of Mr. Cheers on July 10 and had developed the fever on July 24, fifteen days after exposure. Table II describes the cases of thirteen more families in Middlewich, attended by Mr. Taylor. Again, there is remarkable detail in the data. We are told of T. Wolsey, a boatman, from a "very small dirty house," and of J. Archer, from "a remarkably filthy house and filthy family." Table III sets out the number of days between infection and the development of disease. In seventy-two cases they varied from 36 to 76 days.

In analyzing these data Haygarth concluded that out of 202 susceptible individuals, only 19 had escaped infection, so that only 1 in 20 were so lucky.
He pointed out that the "typhous fever" did not present a great problem when
patients were seen in a clear, large, and airy room. He himself, in his more than
thirty-year practice in Chester, had only had an attack of fever on one occasion.

Haygarth went on to make a number of observations. He admitted that
the disease could sometimes be caught suddenly. He thought that prisoners
were less liable to the disease because they were gradually introduced to it. As
to smallpox, he thought it infectious at a greater distance than typhus. He did
not think that clothes exposed to "Typhus miasms" were infectious. He was
not certain how early in the infection it was infectious, but as to the "latent
period" (known to us as the incubation period), out of seventy-two cases it
was less than 10 days in only five cases, less than 17 days in thirteen, between
17 and 33 days in forty-one, and could on occasion be as long as 72 days.

He went on to set out his "Practical Conclusions." There were six of them.
First, medical and clerical staff may safely perform their duties if they follow
his "Rules of Prevention." These, he pointed out, had been communicated to
Thomas Barnard at his request and published by the Society for the Betterment
of the Conditions of the Poor. Second, even nurses may be preserved from infection. Third was the question of schools. Here again, he proposed the removal
of infected individuals to a separate area. In April 1778, for example, Master
Plumbe, "son of a gentleman of fortune in Liverpool," was attacked by fever
at the Rev. Mr. Vanbrugh's school in Chester. He was removed to a separate
chamber and the "Rules for Prevention" were followed. Of thirty-seven boarders, none were infected. By contrast, when a case of fever occurred in a girls'
school of forty pupils, the patient was not isolated and only four girls escaped.
Haygarth considered that the same principles applied equally to other infectious disease, such as smallpox, measles, scarlet fever, chin-cough (whooping
cough), mumps, and so on. His recommendations resulted in the sanatoria that
boarding schools have preserved to this day. Fourth, patients with infectious fevers should never be admitted to hospital wards containing patients with other
disorders. His fifth conclusion was, as he had proposed since his studies of the
population and diseases of Chester nearly thirty years before, that he thought it
essential that when cases of infectious fever occurred in small and dirty houses
the infected persons be removed to a separate building, or to fever wards as
at Chester. He went on to point out that, unlike elsewhere, the fever wards at
Chester had been unopposed when introduced, that they had not excited much
attention for this reason, and that their introduction had been "without noise or
almost without notice." They had therefore not been immediately appreciated,

in contrast to the situation in Manchester, where there had been considerable controversy over the introduction of the House of Recovery. In London, as already noted, there were several who had attempted to follow the Chester example, Dr. Saunders at Guys Hospital, William Heberden at St. George's, as well as Dr. Willan and Dr. Lettsom. His sixth and final practical conclusion concerned the prevention of infectious fevers in the Army and Navy, which he considered could be achieved "in like manner."

Haygarth always expressed his gratitude to those who had helped and supported him. In particular, he thanked his physician colleague, William Currie, and the surgeons to the infirmary, Orred, Morrell, Rowlands, and Freeman. He wished to express, he wrote, his "ever grateful acknowledgement for their uniform encouragement and assistance in the execution of these measures."

There was another comment. He thought that his proposals were as applicable to the army and the navy as they were to civilians. To this end, he was concerned that military tents should be kept as airy as they could be. He proposed that three grooves should be cut at the top of each tent to allow the free passage of air. They were to be covered with a small triangle of cloth so that they would "permit the foul air to escape, and yet to keep out the rain." One soldier commented, after sleeping in such a tent, that "it was a power sweeter in the morning."

Haygarth's conclusion to his *Letter to Dr Percival* read as follows:

> To you this Letter is addressed, as a witness of several transactions which it records, and as a Physician, whose private and professional character has long merited the sincerest regard and esteem of your faithful friend
>
> John Haygarth

In this work, Haygarth also mentioned that on his arrival in Bath he had found that there were attic stories in the infirmary that could with profit be converted into fever wards on the Chester model. There is no evidence that this ever occurred.

Rheumatism

Haygarth then embarked on what was intended to be the first in a series of medical works entitled "A Clinical History of Disease."[228] The first two

---

[228] John Haygarth, *A Clinical History of Disease*, Part 1, *A Clinical History of Acute Rheumatism;* Part II, *A Clinical History of the Nodosity of the Joints* (Bath: R. Crutwell, 1805).

parts, on acute rheumatism and nodosity of the joints, were published in 1805. His experience of the acute condition was based on 170 case histories. He noted that the majority of his patients were women. His main purpose, he wrote, was to explain "why and in what manner and with what effect I have employed the Peruvian Bark of Chinchona [quinine] as a remedy for this fever." This remedy had been recommended to him by Dr. Fothergill and it came in due course to replace bloodletting as a form of treatment. On nodosity of the joints, which he differentiated from other forms of joint deformity, he analyzed 34 out of the 10,549 patients whose illnesses he had recorded during his years in practice in Chester, an incidence of 1 in 310. He clearly distinguished the condition from gout, and from acute and chronic rheumatism. He pointed out that "the nodes, in their gradual progress, sadly embitter the comforts of life but I know of no instance in which they seemed to shorten its duration." The first patient he had seen with this affliction was in fact 93 years old.

The account of the nodes in the fingers that Haygarth gave in his publication had in fact been preceded by a year or two by William Heberden's description of the same condition (De Nodis Digitorum) in his *Medical Commentaries*. These were written in Latin and completed in 1782. They were not published then, but the manuscript was left to his wife after his death in 1801. Heberden wrote, "I desire this book be given . . . for the use of any of my sons who should study physic." His son William, who became a physician, published the work a year later.[229] A translation of his father's description of the knobs on the fingers, which are now called "Heberden's nodes," follows:

> What are those little hard knobs, about the size of a small pea, which are frequently seen upon the fingers, particularly a little below the top, near the joint? They have no connection with the gout, being found in persons who never had it: they continue for life; and being hardly ever attended with pain, or disposed to become sores, are rather unsightly, than inconvenient, though there must be some little hindrance to the free use of the fingers.

Haygarth intended to publish accounts of other disorders but his account of rheumatism and nodosity of the joints was the only one to reach publication. He republished this work more than a decade later, in 1813. As he had done with his *Enquiry*, he circulated his first edition among his

[229] Guilelmi Heberden, *Commentarii de Morborum Historia et Curatione* (London: T. Payne, 1802).

friends, asking them specifically whether they supported the treatment with the bark that he had recommended. This course of action had been suggested by a letter from Sir George Baker, president of the Royal College of Physicians and Physician to their Majesties, who wrote on July 19, 1805, after his work was first published, "You have justified and confirmed the treatment which I have followed for many years." Haygarth specifically directed his queries to friends in London, as it was there that the chinchona bark had been more generally administered than anywhere else. His letter from Bath was dated September 8, 1809. William Heberden, son of Haygarth's old friend, wrote that he used antimonials first, followed by the bark, as his father had taught him. William Saunders thought that the rheumatic fever was "an ague in disguise," for which he used the bark. Robert Willan, now the established founder of the specialty of dermatology, simply wrote, "I can only confirm what you have established." Sir Lucas Pepys told Haygarth, "I place so much confidence in everything that you say, that I have entirely changed my usual method of treating the acute rheumatism, with the greatest success." John Coakley Lettsom was "happy in being on the list of the approvers of your practise." Sir Walter Farquhar had long been a convert to "your mode of treatment," and was particularly successful in his free use of the bark. The last of his replies, written by John Aikin, told him of specific cases in which both he and his son had had success with the use of the bark. It was a roll call of support from some of the most distinguished physicians in the metropolis.

Life in Bath

Problems arose for many citizens following the resumption of hostilities with France in 1803. A year later, Haygarth was writing to solicit the help of the president of the Royal Society in securing the freedom of a young man detained in Geneva by the authorities. He wrote from Bath to Sir Joseph Banks on August 29, 1804,

> I hope that I am not going to take an improper liberty in requesting that you would kindly solicit a particular favour for a very respectable literary friend of mine. Dr Wickham one of Ratcliffes travelling Fellows has been detained a prisoner at Geneva ever since the commencement of the war. He has been *informed that Mr Forbes F. R. S* who was in the same unfortunate situation has obtained his liberty *in consideration of his being a man of science*. It is very well known that the Ratcliffe Travelling Fellows are sent by the University of Oxford to

visit foreign countries for the special purpose of acquiring medical knowledge. Dr Wickham was in France engaged in these important pursuits on the commencement of hostilities. As no Englishman is so generally and so justly known & respected among men of science abroad as well as at home, he has requested the favour of your intercession on his behalf. It is well known that Bonaparte is eminently an encourager of men of science. I can assure you that Dr Wickham is a physician of a most respectable character, likely to become an honour to his profession, being zealously attached to it and endowed with superior abilities. On these considerations. You will, I hope, excuse the liberty of this address, and be the means of my friend's permission to visit Vienna, Berlin, and other parts of Germany & Italy. Such a beneficent assistance would confer the highest obligation on, Dear Sir, your most respectful and faithful humble servant.[230]

Banks, however, could not immediately help. His reply showed that he did not share Haygarth's optimistic view of Bonaparte as a supporter of science. He pointed out that Forbes had been freed on account of his age (he was over 60) rather than as a man of science, and in any case there were other cases that demanded his attention, specifically that of Mathew Flinders, the distinguished navigator and hydrographer, a prisoner of the French in Mauritius. Despite constant pleas to the French authorities, Flinders did not receive his freedom until 1810.

By now Haygarth had lost several more of his contemporaries. William Cullen had died during Haygarth's Chester years, and William Heberden died in London in 1801 at the age of 91, soon after receiving his copy of Haygarth's *Imagination*. Others followed. In 1803, James Currie had a serious recurrence of the pulmonary consumption that was a family legacy. The next year he went to Scotland to put his affairs there in order. He returned to Liverpool in time to go on to Manchester, where Percival, Haygarth's oldest friend and supporter, was seriously ill. Currie stayed at his bedside until his death, after a brief but painful illness, in August 1804. The next year, Currie, himself now mortally sick, traveled to Bath to stay with his daughter at her home in Rivers Street, close to the Royal Crescent. Currie was gratified that his professional colleagues received him "with friendly cordiality." He received invitations to attend a number of Bath conversation parties but only chose to accept that of Haygarth. He would leave his Bath home at 7 p.m. to stay at Haygarth's until 9:00. There he joined fifteen or so others around

[230] Autograph letter, John Haygarth to Sir Joseph Banks, Bath, 29 August 1804, Banks Letters, Mitchell Library, Sydney, New South Wales. The Wickham mentioned by Haygarth may have been H.L.W. Wickham, graduate of Christchurch, Oxford, 1807, son of Sir William Wickham, British diplomat.

116

the fire at the Royal Crescent, sipped tea or coffee, and wondered at the lack of order and the wide range of talk. Currie died later that year.[231] Haygarth was to outlive him by more than twenty years, living on in increasing professional isolation.

---

[231] R. D. Thornton, *James Currie, The Entire Stranger and Robert Burns* (Edinburgh and London: Oliver and Boyd, 1963).

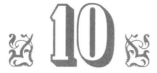

The Pestilential Fever

The Philadelphia Controversy

*H*aygarth continued his close correspondence with American friends such as Waterhouse in Boston. He had been aware of the disastrous epidemics of pestilential (or yellow) fever that had occurred in Philadelphia, most notably in 1793. With his knowledge of the methods he had successfully introduced, it was not surprising that he felt it incumbent on himself to offer advice to the Americans on control of the disease.

Well-meaning in his intentions, he was genuinely surprised when he found himself embroiled in a vigorous controversy over whether the pestilential fever was imported into Philadelphia from abroad—specifically from the West Indies—or whether it originated in the United States. It was an important question for the authorities in the city of Philadelphia, because if it was imported, the correct method of dealing with the disease would be strict quarantine of ships arriving from the Caribbean. On the other hand, if it was due to some form of local putrefaction, then cleaning up the city and its surroundings would be more useful. Haygarth wrote to Waterhouse urging upon him the need to investigate whether the measures taken in Chester and Manchester could be applied to the pestilential fever, though he specifically warned against arguing from analogy.[232] Only the accurate observation of the facts was important. Waterhouse himself had no experience of the disease, as Boston was too far north for the survival of the insect vector ultimately shown to be the transmitter of the disease. He also replied somewhat disappointingly that the American physicians were divided in their opinion respecting yellow fever. Little did Haygarth know how fiercely divided the Philadelphia physicians were.

[232]Weaver, "John Haygarth," 183.

The College of Physicians of Philadelphia had always held the view that the pestilential fever was imported from the West Indies, and they believed further that the disease was contagious.[233] Another group of physicians, led by Benjamin Rush, then noted for the heroic treatment involving massive bleeding and purging that he meted out to his unfortunate victims, argued that there was no evidence of direct contagion and that the disease originated in Philadelphia itself. Rush had a particularly virulent supporter in Charles Caldwell, then a young Philadelphia physician who took inordinate pride in his qualities as an orator. Caldwell had given an address on the subject before the short-lived Academy of Medicine of Philadelphia. He considered that the pestilential fever resulted from the putrefaction of vegetables, a reflection of ancient views on the origins of fever. He ascribed the "whole mischief to a peculiar condition of the atmosphere," which recalled Sydenham and his followers. He went on to say that this was proved by "the great multitude of grasshoppers, flies and muskitos which abounded," an assertion not too far from the truth now that it is known that the yellow fever virus is transmitted by the bite of the mosquito *Aedes Egyptus*.[234]

Haygarth entered the fray at that point. He appended to his *Letter to Dr Percival*, published in 1801, an *Address to the College of Physicians of Philadelphia on the American Pestilence*, in which he strongly supported the views of the college, published in their formal report of 1798, that the pestilential fever was imported.[235] He had in addition had the opportunity of seeing Caldwell's *Address to the Academy*, because he had received a copy from Lettsom, a correspondent of Caldwell. Haygarth did not hesitate to criticize the assertions of Rush and Caldwell.

He also castigated the hypothesis of Noah Webster, one of those to whom Caldwell referred admiringly in his tract, that the great Philadelphia epidemic of 1793 had been associated with natural phenomena such as earthquakes, comets, tornados, and the like. Such weird imaginings would have cut no ice with Haygarth. Webster, America's great lexicographer, was not a medical man. He had a legal background but like many laymen of his time did not hesitate to enter the medical arena. He unhesitatingly supported the idea that the pestilential fever originated in America and was not imported.

---

[233] *Proceedings of the College of Physicians of Philadelphia Relating to the Prevention of the Introduction and Spreading of Contagious Disease* (Philadelphia: Thomas Dobson, 1798).

[234] Charles Caldwell, *A Semi-Annual Oration on the Origin of Pestilential Disease. Delivered before the Academy of Medicine of Philadelphia on the 17th December 1798* (Philadelphia: Thomas and Samuel F. Bradford, 1799).

[235] John Haygarth. Appendix to *Letter to Dr Percival*.

In 1799 he had published a tract (so mercilessly criticized by Haygarth), arguing that it was physical phenomena that preceded and accompanied outbreaks of fever.[236]

In view of his strongly held views on the transmission of infectious fevers, it was not surprising that Haygarth made the very reasonable suggestion that the college should seek to determine just how far distant from an infected person the disease polluted the atmosphere, just as he had done for smallpox and other infectious fevers in Chester. Caldwell, who in the euphoria of those post-Colonial days did not take kindly to an Englishman interesting himself in an "American Disease," was incensed. He wrote a reply to Dr Haygarth's *Letter to Dr Percival and Address to the College of Physicians of Philadelphia* exposing, as he put it, "the medical, philosophical and literary errors of the author and vindicating the right that the Faculty of the United States have to think and decide for themselves respecting the diseases of their country uninfluenced by the notions of the Physicians of Europe."[237] Caldwell's *Address to the Academy* was, perhaps appropriately, dedicated to the same Samuel L. Mitchill, professor in Columbia, New York, whose fertile imagination had suggested that nitrous oxide might be an agent of contagion. It was this concept that had led Humphry Davy to carry out the studies of the effects of breathing nitrous oxide in both animals and man that had shown that the gas was innocuous.

Caldwell's attack on Haygarth was a piece of xenophobic invective that equaled in virulence anything that Tom Paine had written in *Common Sense* at the time of the American Revolution. In three successive sections he sought to destroy Haygarth's character as a scholar, as a philosopher, and as a man of candor and veracity. He concluded with the following severe admonition: "Never again so far forget yourself as to engage in a controversy where genius and science enter the lists; never again dare to approach, with hostile intentions, the temple erected to truth on this side of the Atlantic by the genius of a *Webster*, a *Mitchill* or a *Rush*." Caldwell, who knew that Lettsom had sent a copy of his *Address to the Academy* to Haygarth, later wrote, "By the latter gentleman (Haygarth) it was criticised so unjustly, and under so many misrepresentations of its contents that I replied to his tirade, in a pam-

---

[236] Noah Webster, *A Brief History of Epidemic and Pestilential Disease: with the Principal Phenomena of the Physical World which Precede and Accompany them, and Observations from the Facts stated*, 2 vols. (Hartford: Hudson and Goodwin, 1799).

[237] Charles Caldwell, *A reply to Dr Haygarth's "Letter to Dr Percival on Infectious Fevers and his Address to the College of Physicians of Philadelphia on the Prevention of the American Pestilence"* (Philadelphia: Thomas and William Branford, 1802).

phlet so burning and sarcastic, that he never forgave me, but writhed under the lashing I bestowed on him until the end of his life."[238] Lettsom wrote that he should have treated an older member of the profession with more courtesy, to which Caldwell replied, "When an old man employs language, and perpetrates actions of any sort unworthy of his years, and especially when he violates the truth for the sake of temporarily succeeding in some sinister purpose, he ought for the sake of the example, to be severely rebuked by the young as well as the old." He went on to say that not long afterward Dr. Haygarth died, a fate supposedly meted out to the many opponents he encountered throughout his belligerent career.

Haygarth in fact survived, and he continued to pursue his interest in the pestilential fever. He returned to the subject in 1806 when he wrote a letter from Bath to "The Gentlemen of the College."[239] His letter had been prompted by the further account that the Philadelphia College had recently published supporting its long-held view that the disease was imported.[240] Haygarth was able to inform the college of information he had received in Bath describing the severe outbreak of pestilential fever in Gibraltar and Spain two years before. He referred to his previous *Address*, of 1801, which, he understood, had never reached the college and which, referring to Caldwell, had been, he noted, given so bad a character by the college's opponents "that few people in America had read it." He had prevailed upon Dr. Fellowes, physician to the Forces in Gibraltar and later a physician to the Prince of Wales, to undertake an inquiry into how the pestilential fever was brought into the garrison in 1804. As the college would know, he pointed out, it was the consequence of the fatal error that the disease was not infectious that it rapidly spread, causing in Gibraltar and Southern Spain 12,000 cases of which nearly half were mortal. It was through this outbreak that Samuel Taylor Coleridge passed, mercifully spared, on his way to Malta. Haygarth gave his unequivocal view that he was "clearly convinced that the sphere of infection from the Pestilential Fever is confined to a very narrow distance and that its progress might be effectively prevented by separation, cleanliness and ventilation, exactly in the same

[238] Harriet J. Weaver, *The Autobiography of Charles Caldwell M.D.* (New York: Da Capo Press, 1965).

[239] Autograph letter from John Haygarth to the Gentlemen of the College of Physicians of Philadelphia, Bath, 16 October 1806, from the Library of the College, cited with their kind permission.

[240] Whitfield J. Bell, *The College of Physicians of Philadelphia: A Bicentennial History* (Canton, MA: Science History Publications, 1987), 38.

manner as has for some years been successfully accomplished in regard to Typhus Fever in Chester, Manchester, London and other towns in Britain and Ireland." In this, of course, with no inkling of the insect transmission of infectious disease, he was in error. His utter belief in the correctness of his own ideas illustrates the hazard of attempting a universal syllogism on the basis of a single proposition.

The dispute rumbled on. In 1806 Lettsom attempted to reconcile Haygarth with his Philadelphia critics. Haygarth, now 66 years old, replied uncompromisingly to Lettsom in a letter in which he wrote, "I cannot think that a correspondence with Dr Caldwell would answer any useful purpose." He went on, somewhat portentously, "Truth will at last certainly be discovered. The longer an opinion so manifestly erroneous and as fatally pernicious is defended, the deeper it will fix upon the character of a young physician. Let no man's authority have any influence, but let his own understanding dictate what conclusion ought to be formed from an accurate and faithful report of the facts ascertained by the best evidence." Then, in a perhaps understandable aside, he concluded, " I know too well that the disbelief in the infectious nature of the Pestilential Fever which brought such dreadful destruction at Gibraltar was brought from America."[241] There, so far as Haygarth was concerned, the matter rested. A decade later, however, his views were strongly supported when Sir James Fellowes (1771–1857), as he had now become, published his account of the pestilential disease in Andalusia in 1815.[242] The term "pestilential disease" has, however, to be interpreted with some caution. While it seems clear that the disease in Philadelphia was what would now be known as yellow fever, the epidemic disease encountered by Fellowes may have been a malignant form of typhus.

Meanwhile, Haygarth's American adversary, Charles Caldwell, had, in the words of an American historian, continued his career as a spectacular egoist. Disappointed in his hopes of a professorial chair in Philadelphia, he accepted an invitation to the ill-fated medical school in Kentucky in 1817. He moved reluctantly to Louisville in 1837 and was even more reluctantly evicted from his chair there in 1849 at the advanced age of 77. He died in

[241] Autograph letter, John Haygarth to Dr. Lettsom, Bath 16 October 1806, from the collection of the Wellcome Library for the History and Understanding of Medicine, London.

[242] James Fellowes, *Report of the Pestilential Disease of Andalusia which appeared at Cadiz in the Years 1800, 1804, 1810, and 1813: with an Account of that fatal epidemic as it prevailed at Gibraltar during the Autumn months of 1804; also observations on the remitting and intermittent fever, made at the Military Hospital in Colchester upon the return of the Troops from the Expedition to Zealand in 1809* (London: Longman, Hurst, Rees, Orme and Brown, 1815). See also *DNB*, 18:300.

1853. As Lloyd Stevenson has so cogently put it, he had always been "one of the chief priests of the Great God Blah in an era much given to Blahworship. He talked his life away."[243]

Evidence from the West India Islands

The conclusion of the College of Physicians of Philadelphia that the pestilential fever was imported was now to receive further support from Bath. Haygarth was approached by Colin Chisholm, a physician then living in retirement in Clifton, who had considerable experience of the disease in the West Indies.[244] Chisholm had been physician to His Majesty's Ordnance in the Island of Grenada at a time when the pestilential fever first appeared there in 1793. In that year the ship *Hankey* had arrived from the African coast, its passengers and crew having suffered an appalling mortality during their voyage across the Atlantic. They had sailed from England to the Guinea coast of Africa without any mishap, but as soon as they arrived at the island of Boullam the pestilential fever had broken out among them. They recruited seamen from British navy vessels to replace men they had lost, but they too fell victim to the disease. Crossing the Atlantic, there were deaths virtually every day. By the time they reached Grenada there had been twenty fatalities as well as much sickness. On arrival a friend of the captain went on board; he too perished within a few days. After that one exposure, further cases occurred, the disease having been introduced onto the island by a "negro-wench" who took in washing for the sailors. Soon the disease reached the blacks working on the plantations inland. It is not surprising that Chisholm was at once convinced that it was the ship that had introduced the disease. The disease was not known on the island before that time, making it extremely unlikely that local influences, as argued by Caldwell and his supporters in Philadelphia, could have been responsible.

Chisholm's account of the voyage of the *Hankey* and the ensuing epidemic was described in 1795, when he published his book, *An Essay on the Malignant Pestilential Fever introduced into the West Indian Islands from Boullam on the Coast of Guinea. As it appeared in 1793 and 1794.*[245] He dedicated his

[243] Lloyd Stevenson, introduction to Weaver, *The Autobiography of Charles Caldwell.*

[242] Colin Chisholm (d. 1825), *Oxford DNB;* 11:485–486.

[245] Colin Chisholm, *An Essay on the Malignant Pestilential Fever introduced into the West Indian Islands from Boullam on the Coast of Guinea. As it appeared in 1793 and 1794* (London: C. Dilly, 1795).

work to "The Medical Gentlemen of His Majesty's Navy and Army," as well he might, for he estimated that 200 out of 500 sailors died of the disease during those and later epidemics. His work was republished in Philadelphia in 1799, together with a letter to Professor Whytt in Edinburgh written by John Lining from Charleston, South Carolina, in December 1753. He described epidemics of the pestilential fever in 1733, 1739, 1745, and 1748, conclusively showing that the disease had been imported from the West Indies.[246] Chisholm was again in print two years later, in 1801, when he added *Observations and Facts, tending to prove that the Epidemic existing at Philadelphia, New York &c was the same fever introduced by infection imported from the West India Islands.*[247] This time there were two volumes. His conclusions did not, however, impress those Americans who did not believe that the disease had been imported. In New York, a Dr. Miller wrote a report to the governor of New York State describing the disease that had prevailed in New York in the autumn of 1805, stating unequivocally that "this Malignant Disease had owed its origin to local and domestic causes."[248] Noah Webster also continued in his belief in the domestic origin of yellow fever. In his letters to William Currie of Philadelphia he vehemently opposed Chisholm's concept that the disease had been brought from Africa to the Caribbean and from there to America. He also sought to undermine Chisholm's credibility by attacking the accuracy of his account of the voyage of the *Hankey*.[249]

By now Colin Chisholm had been living in retirement in Clifton for several years. He clearly found a kindred spirit in John Haygarth, for he wrote, "The frequent opportunities you have indulged me in a free and reciprocal communication of sentiment on medical subjects, and more especially that

[246] Colin Chisholm, *An Essay on the Malignant Pestilential Fever introduced into the West Indian Islands from Boullam on the Coast of Guinea. As it appeared in 1793 and 1794. To which is appended a Description of the American Yellow Fever, which prevailed in Charleston in 1748.* (Philadelphia: Thomas Dobson, 1799).

[247] Colin Chisholm, *Observations and Facts, tending to prove that the Epidemic existing at Philadelphia, New York &c was the same fever introduced by infection imported from the West India Islands* (London: J. Mawman, 1801).

[248] Colin Chisholm, *Letter to John Haygarth from Colin Chisholm, author of An Essay on the Pestilential Fever exhibiting further evidence of the infectious nature of this fatal distemper in Grenada in 1793, 4, 5, & 6 and in the United States of America from 1793 to 1805 in order to correct the pernicious doctrine propagated by Dr Edward Miller and other American Physicians related to this destructive Pestilence* (Bath: R. Crutwell, 1809).

[249] Benjamin Spector, *Noah Webster's Letters on Yellow Fever addressed to Dr William Currie*, supplement no. 9 to the *Bulletin of the History of Medicine* (Baltimore: Johns Hopkins University Press, 1947).

most important one, infection, and the propagation of certain types of fever by contagion, leaves me no room to doubt that we think alike on it." In 1809, he published an extended letter to John Haygarth summarizing his experiences. The title of his new work clearly illustrated his purpose: *Letter to John Haygarth MD FRS from Colin Chisholm MD FRS, Author of An Essay on the Pestilential Fever exhibiting further evidence of the infectious nature of the fatal distemper in Granada in 1793, 4, 5 & 6 and in the United States of America from 1793 to 1805 in order to correct the pernicious doctrine propagated by Dr Edward Miller and other American Physicians related to this destructive Pestilence.*[248] Chisholm's comprehensive account of the transmission of the disease in the Caribbean from ship to island and from ship to ship was compelling evidence of the infectious nature of the disease. Specifically, Chisholm republished his account of the disease as it crossed the Atlantic from the West African Coast in the ship *Hankey*, quoting directly from the ship's log, which recorded the appalling mortality among both passengers and crew during their unhappy voyage. His *Letter* gave strong support to Haygarth's views and to the report of the College of Physicians of Philadelphia.

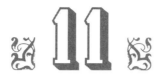

Philanthropy

The Education of the Children of the Poor: A National Church Scheme

*A*s John Haygarth reached his 70s he became progressively less committed to medical matters. He occasionally responded to requests for advice, as when, in March 1808, he was consulted about the case of "my young friend, Mr Crosse." The remedies that had been employed seemed to "have had a salutary effect." Haygarth gave advice on diet, prescribed anodynes for pain, and warned particularly of the danger of catching cold. The young man was never to use violent exercise, a caution he considered "of great importance for the preservation of his health." The outcome of this consultation is not recorded.[250]

Haygarth now became increasingly involved in philanthropic activities. In 1808, he returned to the question of the education of the children of the poor that had so occupied him during his years at Chester. Just as he had sought to extend his Chester studies on smallpox to the establishment of a national institution for the eradication of smallpox, so now he was considering how the expansion of charity schools for the poor on the model of the Chester Blue-Coat school could be extended nationwide.

At that time there was great interest in the question of what sort of education was suitable not only for young men of the monied classes but also for

[250] John Haygarth, autograph letter, in *Letter Book of William Collyns, 1787–1822*, Library of the Royal College of Physicians of London.

the children of the poor. Locke's book *Some Thoughts concerning Education* had a major influence on educational thinkers. By the end of the eighteenth century, Richard Lowell Edgeworth, member of the Lunar Society of Birmingham and father of the novelist Maria Edgeworth, wrote *Practical Education* with his daughter, which emphasized practical, technical, and scientific education.[251] Edgeworth's son-in-law, the Bristol physician Thomas Beddoes, had published his *Extract of a letter in Early Instruction*; Beddoes was a protagonist of universal education.[252] At the same time there were men such as Joseph Lancaster who were developing educational facilities for the poor, specifically using senior pupils to undertake the education of their younger fellows. Hannah More was one of the pioneers of Sunday Schools. She too sought to encourage the education of the children of the poor. Very much involved in the Sunday School movement of that era, she extended her activities to day schools. At first she, with her sister, attracted attention by arguing that the schools would teach children not to rob orchards, but they soon had 500 children being schooled at Cheddar, where they held evening meetings for the parents. Hannah More's views on education were not in any way advanced. She taught the Bible and the catechism and "such coarse works as may fit them for servants." In later years she was to oppose the doctrine that the poor were to be made "scholars and philosophers."[253]

Haygarth had had to face the question of education for his sons. For the well-to-do there was at that time the choice of schools such as Eton, Winchester, and Harrow. Haygarth chose Rugby for his own children, his older son William entering the school at the age of thirteen in 1797 and the younger John two years later at the same age.[254] Rugby had been founded in 1587 and was one of the emerging public schools of modern England, providing instruction for the upper classes and for an increasing bourgeoisie. It had not yet been transformed by the pioneering efforts of Thomas Arnold, who did not arrive as headmaster until 1828.

Haygarth now wrote a long letter to the Right Reverend Bishop Porteus, his old friend from Chester who had strongly supported him in extending the education available at the Blue-Coat School to a far wider group of pupils than

[251] R. L. Edgeworth and M. Edgeworth, *Practical Education,* ed. Jonathan Wordsworth (Poole: Woodstock, 1996).

[252] Dorothy A. Stansfield, *Thomas Beddoes, M.D., 1766–1808: Chemist, Physician, Democrat* (Dordrecht, Boston, Lancaster: D. Riedel, 1984). See also Thomas Beddoes, *Extract of a Letter on Early Instruction, particularly that of the Poor,* 1792.

[253] Hannah More (1745–1833), *Oxford DNB;* 39:39–46.

[254] Information kindly provided by the librarian, Temple Reading Room, Rugby School.

the previous charity school allowed.[255] Porteus was now bishop of London, a more influential diocese than provincial Chester. He had a long-standing interest in education. He strongly supported the Sunday School movement and had recently published a letter to the authorities in the West Indies endorsing plans for the education of the children of negroes. He had sent a copy to Haygarth, for which he received thanks. But Haygarth's main purpose was, as he stated in the title of his letter, to propose a plan that might give a "Good education to all the Poor Children in England." It was a scheme that should in his view come under the aegis of the Church of England. Although many of his friends were dissenters, for example, the Unitarians Drs. Currie and Percival, he was concerned that "various classes of dissenters, with enthusiastic diligence, are teaching the lower classes of children to read, &c in great numbers with great diligence." It was a development he did not favor, for he believed, as did others, that the clergy or the government should take measures to prevent "the adoption [by dissenters] of religious doctrines which in both a religious and a moral point of view are of so highly pernicious a nature."

Haygarth argued that Chester's example of seeking to provide an education for all poor children could with benefit, and at very little cost, be adopted throughout the major towns in England. He entreated the bishop to form a general plan that would come under the guidance and direction of the ministers of religion throughout the land. It was likely that such a proposal would be strongly supported in Ireland. He thought that the king might be persuaded to appoint as bishops individuals who had been most effective in promoting such measures, and that legislation might also prove beneficial. He cited in support of his views the general approval that had been given to Sunday Schools, pioneered by Robert Raikes[256] and strongly supported by bishops such as Porteus, as well as by Hannah More. Haygarth was not alone in his proposals. In that same year, 1808, Andrew Bell[257] had published his pamphlet, *A Sketch of a National Institution for training the Children of the Poor.* At the same time, Herbert Marsh,[258] Lady Margaret's professor of divinity at Cambridge, had preached a sermon in St. Paul's entitled "The National Religion: The Foundation of National Education."

---

[255] Haygarth, *A Private Letter to Dr Porteus.*

[256] Robert Raikes (1736–1811), *Oxford DNB;* 45:804–805. An independent minister and educationalist, Raikes was a promoter of Sunday Schools. He was born and died in Gloucester

[257] Andrew Bell (1753–1832), in *Oxford DNB;* 4:900–905. Founder of the Madras system of education.

[258] Herbert Marsh (1757–1839), *Oxford DNB*; 36:797–801.

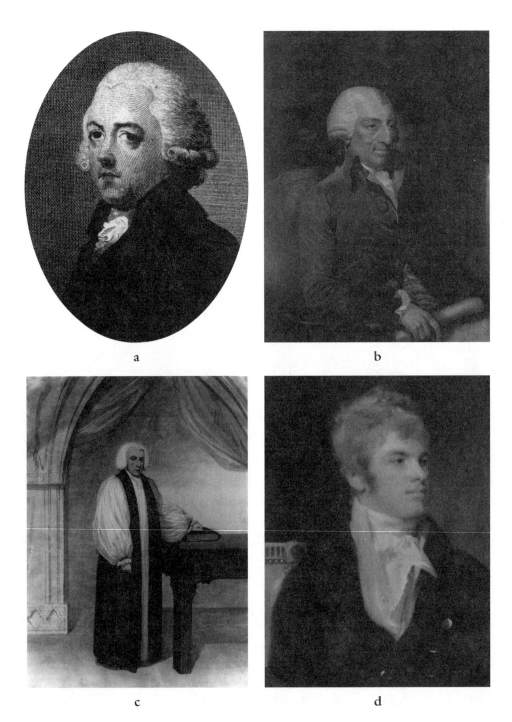

a

b

c

d

Haygarth's letter to the bishop was private and so not published at once. The bishop replied from Fulham House on July 9, 1808. He had received "your most excellent Letter, which displays in a very strong light that comprehensive mind, that indefatigable benevolence and that ardent zeal for promoting the welfare of mankind in various ways, by which you so eminently distinguished yourself when I had the happiness of your acquaintance at Chester."[255] But the bishop was ailing, and his present state of health could in no way permit him to undertake the task of promoting Haygarth's plan. He promised, however, to put the letter into the hands of some of the leading men in the management of charity schools in the capital, and thought too that it would be even better if 50 or 100 copies of Haygarth's letter were printed and he would then undertake to "disperse" them to people who might be able to facilitate the proposals. Porteus did not live to see the outcome of these proposals. He died later that same year.

A year later Haygarth sent a copy of his *Letter to Dr Porteus* to the Right Reverend Dr. Henry William Majendie,[259] now bishop of Chester and Bangor. Majendie, who had been impressed by the achievements of the Blue-Coat School in Chester after his arrival there, strongly supported Haygarth's plan and thought that schools in every parish should be placed under the aegis of established clergymen who would report regularly to the diocese. He thought too that Haygarth's proposals should be submitted at once to the archbishop of Canterbury, who was at that very moment engaged in "methodising a System of Education for the Poorer Orders, to be submitted to the wisdom of Parliament."[260] The archbishop was Charles Manners-Sutton, and it was he who in October 1811 chaired the meeting that led to the foundation of the "National Society."[261] The aim of the society was to

[259] Henry William Majendie DD (1754–1830), who was of Hughenot extraction, followed Porteus as bishop of Chester and Bangor. He was known for his portly figure and the seriousness of his demeanor. He was strong supporter of Sunday Schools in his diocese.

[260] Information kindly provided by Gabriel Linehan, Lambeth Palace Library, London.

[261] H. J. Burgess and P. A. Welsby, *A Short History of the National Society 1811–1961* (London: National Society, 1961).

FIG. 7a. William Falconer;
  b. John Howard, holding a plan of a lazaretto *(Both courtesy of the Wellcome Library, London.)*
  c. Bishop Bielby Porteus;
  d. The Third Marquis of Lansdowne *(Both courtesy of the National Portrait Gallery, London)*

place a church school in every parish throughout the land. Whether a copy of Haygarth's letter ever found its way into the hands of the founders of the society is uncertain; no copy has been preserved in the Archbishop's Library at Lambeth Palace.

Haygarth's letter was not published until 1812, when it was printed by Crutwell together with the replies from the bishop of London and from bishop Majendie. The documents illustrate Haygarth's strong affiliation with the tenets of the Church of England. His piety was also attested by the family prayer he now offered to the bishop, to be "solemnly pronounced by a parent, or even by a child, every Sunday evening at least, before going to bed, to the whole family upon their knees, by all ranks of people."[262] Brought up in this way, by a father so devoted to his church, it was not surprising that Haygarth's son John became a clergyman.

The Provident Institute at Bath for Savings

During Haygarth's lifetime it was the philanthropically minded well-to-do in society who did so much to establish institutions and organizations that were to benefit their fellow citizens, particularly the poor. As has been described, groups of like-minded individuals would come together to sponsor some specific cause. This was how the new voluntary hospitals and dispensaries were founded, as well as such ventures as Haygarth's smallpox society in Chester. The Houses of Recovery that owed so much to Haygarth's pioneering work in Chester were also established in this way. At the same time, certain societies became vehicles for philanthropic endeavors. The Society for the Propagation of the Christian Gospel, founded to counter error and ignorance through the provision of bibles, and the Society for Bettering the Condition of the Poor belong to this era. But there was another venture to which Haygarth made an important contribution: the founding of savings banks for the benefit of the poor and the encouragement of the thrifty and industrious.[263]

For the poor in Haygarth's time there was no way savings could be safely preserved. The banks would not accept small deposits, and in England they paid no interest. What could the average laborer or those in service at the great houses do? Some would store coins in stockings or in boxes under

---

[262] Haygarth, *A Private Letter to Dr Porteus.*

[263] H. Oliver Horne, *A History of Savings Banks* (Oxford: Oxford University Press, 1947).

beds. Others might have a hiding place up the chimney. But for the thrifty there was always the hazard of burglary, sometimes with fatal results, and the ever-present tricksters who sought to separate those known to have some savings from their money. Friendly Societies had existed since the beginning of the eighteenth century, but they were essentially designed to provide support for workingmen when they were sick or aged and did not provide facilities for savings.

Perhaps the first person to set up a savings bank was the remarkable Quaker lady, Priscilla Wakefield, who founded the Tottenham Benefit Bank in 1804 to receive the savings of all and sundry. Any sum from a shilling upward could be deposited and interest was paid at 5 percent. It was a small venture that did not last, but it was probably the first. George Rose suggested in later years, incorrectly as it turned out, that it was the Society for Bettering the Condition of the Poor that first suggested the idea of savings banks. In fact, its major contribution, no mean one, was to circulate information about the early experiments with savings banks to people who had the means or inclination to make practical use of the information.

It was, however, in Scotland that savings banks that endured were established. A small savings bank was started in West Calder in Midlothian in 1807 by the Rev. John Muckersy, but Henry Duncan, minister of the small parish of Ruthwell near Dumfries, is universally acknowledged to be the "Father of Savings Banks." Duncan was undoubtedly influenced by John Bone, who had published a series of pamphlets between 1805 and 1807. The title of his tract on "tranquillity" indicated his intentions: *The Principle and Regulation of Tranquillity; an Institution commenced in the Metropolis for encouraging and enabling industrious and prudent individuals to provide for themselves and thus effecting the gradual abolition of the Poor's Rate whilst it increases the comforts of the Poor*. He argued that "a Bank should be opened to receive the earnings of the youth of both sexes who have no dependence but their labour and economy, and to return to them on the day of their marriage with the interest and premiums proportioned to the amount."[264]

Henry Duncan was a man of remarkable energy and ability. In 1809 he founded the *Dumfries and Galloway Courier*, becoming its first editor, so that he had the opportunity of propagating many of his thoughts through its columns. In Ruthwell there was a Friendly Society that had been set up in 1796, but it was in a poor way. So, in 1810, Duncan founded the Ruthwell Savings Bank in a small cottage that is there to this day, now preserved as a museum.

[264] George Duncan, *Memoir of the Rev. Henry Duncan of Ruthwell* (Edinburgh: William Oliphant, 1848).

Deposits were received of between 1 shilling and 10 pounds and interest was paid at 4 percent. The money was banked with the British Linen Company, which generously guaranteed interest at 5 percent so that a small sum was available for expenses. The management of the bank was extremely elaborate and Duncan had his critics, but he confounded them when deposits rose to £151 in the first year, then in successive years to £176, £241, and £922. By the end of 1814 they amounted to £1,164. Duncan claimed this achievement as "an astonishing success."[264]

In Bath, John Haygarth was aware of the developments in Ruthwell. In fact, Henry Duncan may well have been known to him. The Duncan family were close kinsmen of the Curries, and Haygarth's Liverpool friend James Currie, originally from Dumfries, had been instrumental in promoting the interests of Henry Duncan's brothers, George, William, and Robert, as merchants in the city.[265] Furthermore, George Duncan was married to Christian Currie, Dr. Currie's sister. In 1790, before the youthful Henry Duncan had decided to enter the ministry of the Church of Scotland, he had worked for three years in Liverpool at Heywood's Bank, during which time he had lodged with Dr. Currie. It was a period that may well have been useful to him in later years when he came to found the Ruthwell Savings Bank.

In Bath at that time four ladies and four gentlemen founded a society "to enable Servants, in Bath, to preserve what part of their wages they could spare."[266] This small venture was so successful that in 1813 attempts were made to extend the facilities of the society to "all the lower classes of people." A general assembly of citizens was called for March 19, when a committee of thirty-five, "highly respectable for their rank, ability and benevolence," was nominated. During March, April, and May attempts were made to form regulations that would allow the same interest to all, and the opportunity of restoring the sums deposited. But for the moment it was to no avail, for the conditions were found to be utterly impracticable.

John Haygarth then came up with a novel scheme that was not to be a savings bank on the Scottish model, but a provident institution.[266] Because the English banks would not pay interest on deposits at a rate that would attract depositors, there had to be another solution. There were three ways in which the Bath group could proceed. First was the option of personal guarantors, never a starter because none would be so injudicious as to hazard their

[265] Christopher C. Booth, "Curries and Duncans in Dumfriesshire," *Proceedings of the Dumfriesshire and Galloway Natural History and Archeological Society* 77 (2003): 211–227.

[266] John Haygarth, *Explanation of the Principle and Proceedings of the Provident Institute at Bath for Savings* (Bath: R. Crutwell, 1816).

personal fortune in this way. Second, they could follow the Scottish example, investing the deposits in funds that would offer a rate of interest slightly less than that obtained from the investments. The third proposal, put forward by Dr. Haygarth, was to transfer to depositors the risks of fluctuation in the funds by making them proprietors of stock to the extent of their deposits.

Haygarth's proposal was set out in his own words in his *Explanation*. The argument ran as follows:

> That each deposit into the Provident Fund shall be made in even pounds. That a Table should be calculated, to determine how much Stock the Deposit has purchased, according to the variations of the 3 per cents, from £50 to £100, (and so of other stocks,) at the time when it was invested in the Funds: That in another Table or Column shall be calculated what Dividend will be due upon the said Stock: That four-fifths of this Dividend shall be given to the Depositor, and one fifth reserved to pay expenses: That a Certificate be given by the Actuary to the person who deposits the money, stating what Stock is purchased with the said deposit, according to the rate calculated in the Tables, and what is the sum arising from four-fifths of the Dividend, which the Depositor is annually to receive. That the annual payments shall be endorsed on the certificate: That after the Stock is sold, the Depositor shall receive the full price of it in money without any expense: That the certificate is then to be given up to the Actuary, and cancelled.

This was put to the consideration of the committee, and it is to Haygarth's credit that his recommendations were at once accepted. It is clear from his writings that Haygarth, perhaps once more using his mathematical knowledge or more probably his experience from managing his own affairs, had a detailed understanding of stock and its fluctuation at that time. He made a careful assessment of the potential effects of variations in the value of stock and pointed out,

> Since the commencement of the Provident Institution, the 5 per cents have varied from 95 to 84. In the last column of the Table of Stock, it appears, that the year's income at £95 was 10d in the pound, or 4l. 3s. 4d. per cent., and at £84 was 11 1/2d. in the pound, or 4l. 15s. 10d. per cent. This income will always remain the same, as long as the money remains invested, whatever may be the variation in the price of Stock.

The Bath Provident Institution was opened on January 17, 1815, and the regulations were published by Haygarth. There was a formidable committee. The patron was the Marquis of Lansdowne,[267] son of the Earl of Shelburne, later the first marquis, who had befriended Haygarth's American friend Arthur Lee in London half a century before. His son was perhaps a particularly appropriate choice, as he had been a youthful chancellor of the exchequer in Lord Grenville's "Administration of all the Talents" in 1806. There were eight trustees, including four members of parliament, George Rose, statesman and philanthropist, Lord John Thynne, Sir J. C. Hippersley, and Colonel Gore Langton. The managers, headed by the mayor of Bath, numbered thirty and were headed by "John Haygarth M. D. F. R. S." It was an immediate success. Deposits during the first year amounted to £4,000, and by 1817 the figure had increased to £17,000.

Banks on the Haygarth model came to be established throughout England, the most influential being the Provident Institution for the Western Part of the Metropolis, opened on Panton Street, Haymarket, on April 15, 1816. The initiative for this development came from the Society for Bettering the Condition of the Poor. There was a distinguished board of trustees and managers, and the president was the Duke of Somerset. The vice presidents included twenty peers, among them the royal Dukes of Kent and Sussex. There were other provident banks on the Haygarth model that were established in the metropolis, including both the London and Bloomsbury Provident Banks. The movement soon spread to the provinces, where similar banks were set up at Southampton, Exeter, and Norwich.

Haygarth paid fulsome tribute to those who had particularly helped him in his endeavors: William Davis, Webbe Weston, and a Colonel Enys. Haygarth recorded that the colonel, whose gout had necessitated his retirement from the army to the healing waters of Bath, was assured by a fellow officer, "You, perhaps, have done as much service for our Country by your labour in forming and executing a Provident Institution, as if you had commanded and led into battle one of the grand divisions of the British Army at Waterloo."[268]

There is little doubt that the savings bank movement was linked in the public mind with other philanthropic and humanitarian movements. As the *Sheffield Mercury* of December 5, 1818 put it,

> As the practice of vaccination bids fair to eradicate the most loathsome and destructive diseases from the earth;—as the establishment of Houses of Recov-

[267] Henry Petty-Fitzmaurice (1780–1863), *Oxford DNB;* 19:900–904. Third Marquis of Lansdowne. Only son by his second marriage of William Petty, second Earl of Shelburne and first Marquis of Lansdowne. Educated at Edinburgh University. Politician and statesman.

[268] Haygarth, *Explanation*, 13.

ery are likely in time to extinguish the infection of fever in our cities and large towns;—as the institution of the Bible Society tend to eradicate error and ignorance from the world;—so the establishment of Savings Banks may ultimately tend to banish poverty and wretchedness from society.

The article concluded,

At some remote age, when the historian of England is relating the glories and exploits of the eighteenth century, he will dwell with particular pleasure on the origin of those improvements, which are probably destined to effect important changes in the condition of the human race, and which indeed will reflect higher honour on our island than the most brilliant successes on sea or on shore.[269]

John Haygarth could have claimed, though he never did, that he had played an important role in those developments.

[269] Horne, *A History of Savings Banks,* 13.

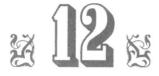

The Last Years

The Move to Swainswick

By 1812, Haygarth's sons were becoming established in their future careers. The elder, William, now 28 years old, had graduated from Cambridge in 1805 and in 1810 obtained a traveling fellowship from the university and departed for a protracted journey to Greece.[270] He was to embark on the uncertainties of a literary and artistic career. John, graduate of Cambridge in 1808, was 26 and had decided on the security of the church.[271] He became a deacon at Winchester in 1809 and in July 1810 married Sophia Poulter, daughter of the Edmund Poulter of Winchester. In November he was ordained priest at Gloucester. The following year his first son, John Sayer Haygarth, was born. In 1814, John Haygarth Jr. was to become rector of Upham, in Hampshire, where he remained until his death forty years later. There is a tablet to his memory in the church there.

William's life was to be more flamboyant. He was a witness at his brother's marriage in July 1810 but set off for Greece soon afterward, taking the sea route by Gibraltar and Malta. He traveled widely in Greece, meeting and dining with Byron in Athens. He left for home in early 1811, was in Malta by the spring, and off the coast of Gibraltar in June. For more than a decade the Royal Crescent had been home to him. Now, on his return from his travels, he found that his family were to move.

In the summer of 1812, the Haygarths moved to Lambridge House, in the parish of Swainswick, although the doctor retained his ownership of the

---

[270] J. J. Venn, *Alumni Cantabrigiensis*, part 2, vol. 3 (Cambridge: Cambridge University Press, 1947), 301.

[271] Ibid.

house in the Royal Crescent until 1819.[272] His new home was a spacious house on the south side of the London Road as it leaves Bath. Swainswick, a small village with an ancient Norman church set among rolling hills, must have reminded him of home. Now in his early 70s, perhaps he found the country church a more congenial place to worship than the center of fashionable Bath. Perhaps he was seeking an appropriate resting place for his old bones when the time came. His daughter Mary, with no suitor apparent, stayed on with her parents.

Lambridge House soon became the center of Haygarth family life. Son John's second and third children, Sophia Mary born in 1813 and Sarah Vere born three years later, were both christened at Swainswick. William seems to have stayed with his parents for at least some of the years after his visit to Greece. In 1813, he was writing his book on Greece, a poem in blank verse, while at Lambridge House.[273] It was published in 1814, and attracted variable reviews. In 1816, after the end of the Napoleonic wars when it again became possible to travel on the continent, he visited Italy. He was also in Geneva when Byron and Shelley were there but there is no indication that he met them, nor any evidence that he attended the soirees of his father's correspondent, Louis Odier. He was in Bath a year later when Fanny Burney recalled meeting him at a party hosted by Miss Harriet Maltby, one-time neighbor of the Haygarths at No. 22, The Royal Crescent. Fanny wrote in a letter that she had met "a young man who is celebrated for a poem called 'Greece,' which he has published. . . . He added, however, nothing to the entertainment of the evening, for he avoids making a parade of his travels and knowledge by a contrary extreme; that of a reserve that leads him only to speak when spoken to, and only to answer concisely to the propositions presented to him; so that all conversation drops with his first answer, or is to be renewed at the expense of a fresh interrogatory."[274] William seems, however, not to have shunned the social scene in Bath. There were others who remembered him. The physician son of his father's old friend Thomas Percival, Edward Percival, was then practicing in Bath.[275] He was almost an exact contemporary of the Haygarth boys and may have known them from

---

[272] The date of the move to Lambridge House is documented by entries in the Rates and Poors, as well as in legal and family documents. Information provided by Professor Stella Miller-Collett, personal communication.

[273] William Haygarth, *Greece, a poem . . . with notes, classical illustrations and sketches of the scenery* (London: Bulmer, 1814).

[274] *The Diary and Letters of Madame D'Arblay,* edited by her niece (London: Henry Colburn, 1854), 204.

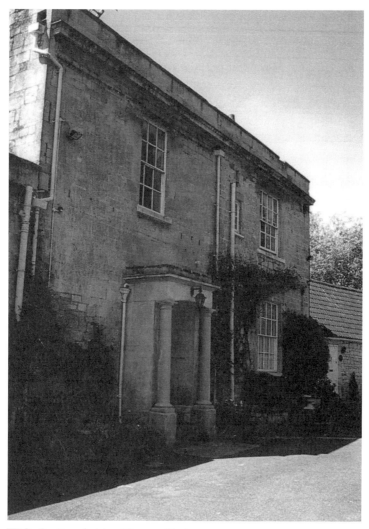

FIG. 8. Lambridge House, Bath
(Photograph by the author.)

[275] See Venn, *Alumni Cantabrigensis.* Edward Percival (1783–1819) was the third son of Thomas Percival of Manchester. He graduated in medicine at Trinity College, Dublin, in 1810. After practicing in Dublin for some years, he moved to Bath, where he practiced until his premature death in 1819.

their early years. He spoke about William Haygarth favorably, "as one who improved on acquaintance, as well his book. I collected that he was a calm, dignified sort of Gentleman, quite a Doric pillar."[276]

As is the lot of those who live to a great old age, however, John Haygarth's last years were darkened by bereavement. At the end of 1815, just after he had published his work on the provident institute at Bath, his wife of forty years, the mistress of his household for so long, died at Lambridge House. Her death was sudden. Hester Piozzi wrote to a friend that in Bath at that time "sudden death was never so frequent." Mrs. Haygarth, she recorded, was only "ten or twelve hours bad."[277] Nevertheless, as a widower Haygarth seems to have lived a life of contentment with his daughter Mary. In 1818, Maria Edgeworth (1767–1849), the popular novelist, wrote to tell a friend that she had breakfasted with

> Dr Haygarth and Miss Haygarth sister and father to that Mr Haygarth who wrote the poem of Greece which I talked of so much to you. Dr and Miss Haygarth are both well informed and agreeable and the family seemed much attached. . . . We saw all Mr Haygarth's drawing taken in Italy–Greece–Switzerland–The Tyrol &c. They are admirable sketches. Mr Haygarth himself was not at home or rather he was at his own home—has settled on his own estate in Hampshire. I hope we may meet him when or if we go to London.[278]

Maria was the daughter of Richard Lovell Edgeworth (1744–1817) and the sister of Anna, the wife of Thomas Beddoes, with whom Humphry Davy had worked at Bristol. Davy called Anna "the best and most amiable woman in the world." Maria's cooperation with her father on the book *Practical Education* may well have been a topic of conversation that morning. Maria Edgeworth clearly had a high opinion of William Haygarth's literary work. In a letter to her friend and fellow author Anna Barbauld, sister of the doctor's old friend John Aikin, she wrote of William's poem *Greece*: "I think if he cultivates his interests, he may either become a fine historian, or a fine tragedian." Anna replied, "My brother is delighted that you are pleased with Mr Haygarth's Poem, for the author is the son of a

[276] Letter from Charles St. George to his mother Melesina Trench. Hampshire Record Office, 23 M 93/15/1/113. Personal communication from Professor Stella Miller-Collett.

[277] *Gentleman's Magazine* 1 (1816): 87. See also Edward A. Bloom and Lillian D. Bloom, eds., *The Piozzi Letters: Correspondence of Hester Lynch Piozzi, 1784–1821 (Formerly Mrs. Thrale)*, vol. 5, *1811–1816* (Newark: University of Delaware Press, 1989–99), 435, 437.

[278] Maria Edgeworth, *Letters from England 1813–1844*, ed. Christine Colvin (Oxford: Clarendon Press, 1971), 85.

very intimate friend of his, a Physician." No doubt these views were conveyed to the proud parent.

In 1820, John Haygarth would have been saddened to hear of the death in Sedbergh of his old teacher, John Dawson. Geologist Adam Sedgwick, son of Richard Sedgwick, vicar of Dent, had in fact been brought into the world at the Dent vicarage by John Dawson. He was to be the Woodwardian Professor of Geology at Cambridge and had been a pupil of Dawson, just as Haygarth and his father were in the summer of 1756. He has left a lively account of his revered teacher in old age. He described him as

> Simple in manner, cheerful and mirthful in temper, with a dress approaching that of the venerable old Quakers of the Dales, yet did he bear at first sight a very commanding presence . . . his powerful projecting forehead and well-chiselled features might have implied severity had not a soft radiant benevolence played over his fine old face.[279]

Sedgwick saw Dawson just before he died. His mind by then had become clouded and confused, yet as happens so often in old age, he had moments of clarity that surprised his visitors. Sedgwick recorded that although Dawson's daughter, his prop and solace in those last years, had warned him that he would not be able to sustain any long or connected conversation, he "lighted up, talked of old times and early studies, and then, with all his former earnest simplicity of expression and clearness of thought, he spoke of the introduction of the powerful French mathematical analysis into the Cambridge course." Dawson told his old pupil that he was "a feeble old man, and my days are nearly numbered."[279] It was the last flickering of his intellect, for when Sedgwick saw him later that same day his mental power was gone and he had no memory of what had passed between them. Dawson died soon after this last visit, at the age of 86. He was buried at the parish church at Sedbergh, where his ex-students, many now distinguished men, erected a marble bust to his memory. It stands high on the south side of the nave.

Within a year Haygarth was to lose a faithful and affectionate servant. Hannah Beswick had joined the Haygarth family in Chester in 1784, the year the doctor extended his property on Foregate Street. She had moved with the family to the Royal Crescent and then with her aging master to Lambridge House. She died on December 29, 1821, at the age of 72 and

---

[279] Adam Sedgwick, *Supplement to the Memorial to the Trustees of the Cowgill Chapel* (Cambridge: Cambridge University Press, 1870).

was buried at Swainswick, where Haygarth erected a simple stone to her memory, paying tribute to the thirty-seven years she had served his family. Three years later he was to lose his old friend of student days, William Falconer. He died at his house in the Circus at Bath on August 31, 1824, at the age of 80. He was buried at Weston, near the city.

By now his son William was mortally sick. William's literary career had been moderately successful. He had bought an estate at Holly Hill in Sussex in 1818 and married Frances Parry (1794–1886) at St. George's, Hanover Square, a year later. His first son Francis was christened at Swainswick on May 12, 1820. Another son, Henry William, also christened at Swainswick, was born in 1821, and in 1823 there were twin girls, Charlotte Melissa and Isabel Mary. They were born precipitously in an inn in Marlborough, as their parents were making their way to their grandfather's home at Swainswick. The twins were christened there on April 9, but sadly both died within three months. Disaster continued to haunt William's family. By November he himself was seriously ill.[280]

John Haygarth, however, lived on. He seems to have retained both his health and his mental faculties until the end. In 1823, at the age of 83, he wrote to his nephew at Badgerdub in Garsdale, "I feel few infirmities but deafness."[281] He found solace in his family. The christening parties for his grandchildren at Lambridge House and the visits of his sons must have given him great pleasure. In the autumn of 1823 the old man wrote, presumably soon after the twins had arrived, that "William's family have resided with us some weeks. He has two sons and two daughters who have enjoyed perfect good health from their birth. My son John's eldest son [John Sayer] is here at school, and though not twelve years old is very forward in Greek and Latin and various kinds of knowledge; his three sisters are advancing in their education entirely to our satisfaction. My sons and daughter enjoy good health."[281] It was not so for long. William's twins died soon after their grandfather's letter, and by early 1824 William's friends, concerned about his health, were writing that he was "pale, emaciated, eager and hollow-eyed."[280] Supposedly it was consumption. The invalid went to Brighton for a while and in December was well enough to buy Tilgate Manor in Sussex. By April, however, his position was described as "precarious" and he died at

[280] Melesina Trench, letter to her son Chester St. George, February 26, 1824. Hampshire Records Office, 23 M 93/30/1/113. Personal communication from Professor Stella Miller-Collett.

[281] George H. Weaver, "John Haygarth: Portrait, Letter and Descendants," *Bulletin of the Social History of Medicine Chicago* 4 (1928–1935): 264–267.

Epsom in September 1825 when his wife was pregnant with their last child. Arthur was born in 1826, after his father's death. His baptism duly took place at Swainswick, but it must have been an occasion of mixed emotions for the old doctor and his remaining family.

Return to Garsdale

In those last years, Haygarth returned to his roots. He kept in close contact with his nephew James Haygarth at Badgerdub in Garsdale. James was the son of Richard Haygarth, tenant of Swarthgill, one of John Haygarth's half-brothers. After the death of Leonard Haygarth in 1802, James's brother William inherited Badgerdub but he had died soon afterward and the property came to James. James seems to have been an erratic figure, fathering an illegitimate child with Martha Inman from nearby Low House. They were to be married twenty-two months later but the entry in the Parish records appears to have been doctored to make it appear that they were married when their child was born. James kept a nature diary intermittently from 1818 until 1834, recording for the most part his memories of the first cuckoo in spring and parties for shooting rooks but also such life events as his acceptance of the office of constable and a burglary at his home.[282]

John Haygarth's main interests in distant Garsdale were the plantations he was creating on the hillsides above the old family home at Swarthgill, the management of his properties, and the provision of Sunday schooling for the young of his native dale. In response to a letter from the doctor from Bath, James referred to "your enemies in the Plantation ie of the Mice," which were increasing.[281] It was to be a recurring problem, as was the difficulty faced by the workmen in clearing the grass from the roots of the trees. But there was also the question of the Sunday School. Haygarth and his daughter were concerned about the importance of propagating useful knowledge among the poor inhabitants of Garsdale. James responded to the doctor's enquiries by telling him that there were sixty-eight pupils attending on Sundays, but many were "devoid of prayer books." There were three teachers: "Mr Thos Harrison has the leading class, Saml Cooper the next and James Haygarth the little ones."[283] He pleaded with his uncle for

[282] Kevin J. Lancaster, "The Nature Diary of James Haygarth of Badgerdub," *The Sedbergh Historian* 2 (1991): 28–39.

[283] Autograph letter, James Haygarth to his uncle, John Haygarth, 30 November 1819, from the Badgerdub papers, in the possession of Denise Colton.

help with the prayer books, but he would take in what subscriptions he could and pay them to Anthony Harrison, who was now Haygarth's steward and living at Swarthgill.

In 1822 Haygarth paid a visit to Garsdale. The visit was recorded by James Haygarth in his nature journal. Dr. John arrived by post-chaise in Sedbergh with his daughter on June 12, and they picked up John Dawson's daughter for the duration of their visit. They were only a day in Sedbergh but it was an opportunity for John Haygarth to meet the new headmaster of Sedbergh School. From 1799 until 1819 William Stevens, sometime chaplain to the Royal Navy, had been headmaster. When he left the school he had only eight day boys and no boarders. It was a situation that had alarmed Haygarth when he wrote his *A Private Letter to Dr Porteus*; he recorded in a footnote to that letter that in 1811 Stevens had only four scholars.[284] William Wordsworth visited Stephens in Sedbergh in 1819. He also was deeply concerned about the state of the school, to which he intended to send his son John. He found Stephens at death's door—he was to die a week later. Wordsworth then enlisted Lord Lonsdale's support in pressuring St. John's College to appoint a more able successor. They selected the 27-year-old Henry Wilkinson, a fine scholar and a second wrangler, as the new headmaster.[285] It was he who brought the school back to life. Haygarth was able to interview him that day in Sedbergh. Perceptively, he wrote later to his steward, Anthony Harrison at Swarthgill, that he "was very much pleased with him, and entertain very confident expectations that under his management Sedbergh School with be restored to great celebrity and usefulness."[286] There were, however, problems that he would face. Haygarth went on,

> But his time and talents will be so fully engaged in his professional duties, that I perceive he cannot have leisure to undertake to teach his ex-scholars, during the holidays, the principles of divinity according to the Church of England. Can his usher conveniently undertake such an office? You have frequently given him a very favourable character. Can he recommend a good master from St Bees for Garsdale School, if none can be found at Sedbergh & if a competent income can be obtained on the plan you proposed?

[284] John Haygarth, *A Private Letter to Dr Porteus*, 5.

[285] Patrick Tolfree, "William Wordsworth's Links with Sedbergh," *Sedbergh Historian* 4, no. 6 (2003): 19–23.

[286] Autograph letter, John Haygarth to Anthony Harrison, "Lambr July 8, 1822," from the archives of Sedbergh School, kindly contributed by Elspeth Griffiths, archivist and librarian.

Haygarth's interview with Wilkinson seems to have been a hurried affair. He asked Harrison to make some apology to Mr. Wilkinson "for the abrupt & intrusive manner in wch I addressed him on various subjects." He had only been able to spare a small portion of his time during a very busy day at Sedbergh.

He went on to Garsdale with Miss Dawson and his own daughter, staying at Garsdale Hall, a Haygarth property then an inn but now descended into disrepair and neglect. He was unimpressed with the state of the turnpike, a road that led from the tollgate in Garsdale over the Pennines to another at Prye House near Hawes in Wensleydale. In Garsdale he had time to discuss the state of his properties with his steward. He also, as he promised later, undertook to pay the expense of a sewing school for girls in the dale. He and his daughter then left for Chester, where they spent three days with friends, driving on from there to Bath. He told Harrison, "We arrived at home on the 2d July, travelling 94 miles on the last day without fatigue."[286] It had been a remarkable trip for the aging physician.

The plantation was, however, a constant concern. After his return to Bath, Haygarth wrote to Anthony Harrison outlining some of his problems. The workman he had employed, he wrote, "had an engagement . . . to cut away the grass growing around the plants that would smother & destroy them, as was the case with the Swarthgill Plantation."[286] The numbers of plants involved was extraordinary. He went on,

> Owing to this neglect and bad management (by the workman) he was put to the expense of supplying 23088 new plants in 1818 & a considerable number in 1817. You will I know take care that the plants are properly cleared from grass according to the planter's obligation & which is so much to his own advantage. By cutting the grass, the myriads of mice in the West Wood may be prevented in the east wood.—Or may they be devoured by a colony of wild cats?

A letter the next year, 1823, written from Bath by John Haygarth to his nephew James at Badgerdub, tells of further tribulations.[287] James had viewed the west wood and had found a deficiency generally of the fifth tree. But, wrote his uncle doctor,

> An oak was to have been planted every 10th tree & an elm &c every 10th. The latter were I believe devoured by the myriads of mice wch infested the planta-

[287] Weaver, "John Haygarth."

tion & their place probably not supplied as they ought to have been. I believe that the oaks were not so generally destroyed. In favourable weather it may be amusing to walk thro' this plantation and to observe the present states & to suggest how any deficiency may be supplied. I shall be much obliged by your information how the oak, larch, fir, ash, elm and any other of them live and grow & which of them are entirely destroyed.

The Sunday School seems to have been progressing well. Through Haygarth's good offices, James Haygarth recorded that prayer books had been "very feelingly procured of the Society for promoting useful knowledge." It was in 1823 that Haygarth sent his portrait to his Garsdale relations. There were problems with the carriage. It went by coach as far as Birmingham but there was then an extra 5 shillings to pay, which the doctor thought too much. The portrait was later given by his descendants to the Chester Infirmary, where he had labored for so long. There the aged Haygarth looks out on the world with serene amiability, a hint of amusement playing around the corners of his eyes.[288]

He was as active as ever. In 1823, the year of Edward Jenner's death, he wrote in a firm strong hand to his successor in Chester, W. M. Thackeray, cousin of the novelist, with questions on "the introduction, progress and extermination of the late typhus contagion imported from Ireland into Chester."[289] He was spared the intellectual decrepitude that so afflicted John Dawson in his last years. In the year of his death he was writing to his nephew James Haygarth enquiring about the state of the "School at Swarthgill." As was his practice, he put a series of queries to his nephew.

[288] In 1931, the portrait was presented by Miss Annie S. Haygarth, a great-granddaughter of John Haygarth, to the Chester Royal Infirmary. See ibid. It hangs today in the postgraduate center of the Countess of Chester Hospital, which has replaced the Chester Infirmary, now closed. Personal communication from Giles R. Young, consultant physician to the hospital.

[289] Autograph letter, John Haygarth to Dr. Thackeray, Lambridge House, 10 May 1823, from the Wellcome Library for the History and Understanding of Medicine. W. M. Thackeray continued Haygarth's interest in infectious disease during his own career in Chester. He was an early member of the Provincial Medical and Surgical Association, the forerunner of the British Medical Association, which was founded in Worcester by Sir Charles Hastings in 1832. On the first anniversary year of the association, Thackeray offered a prize for an essay on a medical subject. There were no takers that year but he then increased the value of his prize to £50. His proposed subject would have been close to Haygarth's heart: "The source of the common contagious fevers of Great Britain and Ireland and the ascertaining of the circumstances which may have a tendency to render them communicable form one person to another." The prize was awarded to a Dr. Davidson of Glasgow in 1840. E. M. Little, *History of the British Medical Association 1832–1932* (London: British Medical Association, 1934).

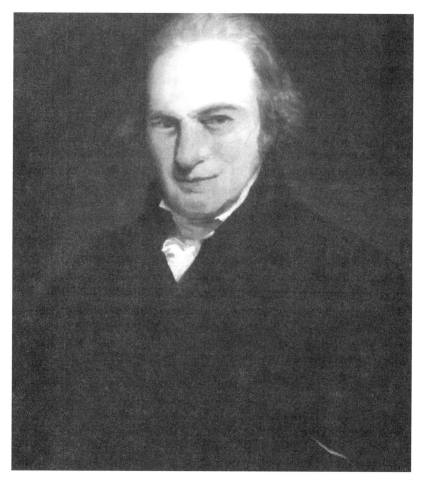

FIG. 9. John Haygarth in old age, artist unknown
(Courtesy of the Countess of Chester Hospital NHS Trust.)

There were nine in all, which James endeavored to answer.[290] He wrote to his uncle that the school "prospers very much." It was open on Sundays but not on weekdays, for "reading writing and spelling." There were forty-seven scholars on Sundays but they lacked "sloping boards." The door, he told his uncle, opened onto the Public Road. It must have been of considerable satisfaction to Haygarth that this, the last of his educational projects, had been a success.

[290] Autograph letter, James Haygarth to his uncle, John Haygarth, 5 January 1827, from the Badgerdub papers. There is a tablet to James Haygarth's memory in the church at Garsdale.

Resting Place at Swainswick

Haygarth died at Lambridge House in early June 1827. He was buried at St. Mary's, the small but beautiful Norman church at Swainswick. The church seems to hide itself from the world, in a hollow reachable only by a single-track lane along which Haygarth would have made his final journey. His tomb carries a simple inscription but on the wall to the left of the nave is a large marble tablet upon which is inscribed,

This monument is erected
In affectionate remembrance of
John Haygarth MD FRS
Late of Lambridge House in the Parish
In public life he may be regarded
As a PHYSICIAN
Who advanced the cause
Of medical science by his writings
And exercised much sagacity
In his treatment of diseases
As a PHILOSOPHER
He is known to have added to the Stock
Of well authenticated facts
Concerning the influence of the mind upon the body
As a PHILANTHROPIST
He was unwearied in his exertions
To diminish the amount of human misery
Active in his endeavours
To spread the blessings of education
Throughout the Land
And ardent in his plans
To increase the comforts of the poor
In private life he was strong
In his domestic attachment
Constant in his friendships
Tender in his sympathy

FIG.10a. St. Mary's Church, Swainswick;
    b. The tomb of John Haygarth *(Both photographs by the author.)*

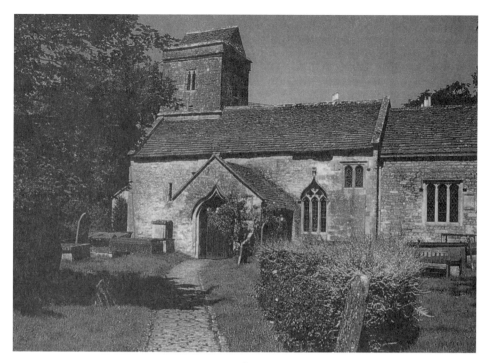

a

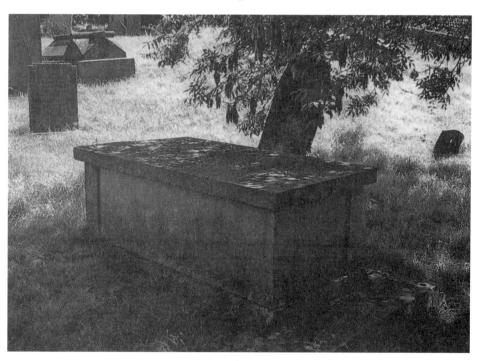

b

151

And abounding in goodwill to all
He died in reliance
On the atoning Blood
Of his Saviour
June 10th 1827
Aged 87 years

Back in his native Garsdale he is remembered by an elegant marble and stone pulpit presented by his granddaughter to the village church where he had worshipped as a boy. The inscription reads, "To the Glory of God and in Memory of John Haygarth MD FRS." At Chester he was remembered by the naming of the old fever ward at the Chester Infirmary, later to be used as a children's ward, the "Haygarth Ward." In addition, for many years the best nurse at the hospital was rewarded with a silver medal known as the Haygarth Medal. To this day there is also a Haygarth Ward at the Royal United Hospital in Bath.

Haygarth's will, dated 1825, was presumably drawn up after the unexpected death of his elder son William that same year.[291] It shows that he now left the major part of his estate to his surviving son John, the rector of Upham. All his silver plate went to his grandson Francis, eldest son of William.[292] There was a trust fund for his daughter Mary, who had cared for him devotedly until the end. It amounted to the remarkable sum of £14,200. The conditions of the will specifically set out how the trust should be apportioned in the event of Mary's marriage and any possible children of such a union. In the event, no suitor for Mary appeared. In 1727, Mary went to live with her brother at Upham, where she died on January 9, 1850, at the age of 72. Tantalizingly, there was no mention in the will of the doctor's papers, nor of the case records he had so carefully amassed during his Chester years. They have simply disappeared.

[291] Olive Haygarth, "The Family History of Dr. John Haygarth," *The Sedbergh Historian* 2, No. 5 (1990):14–18. A copy of his will is preserved at the Public Record Office (PROB11/1731).

[292] Francis Haygarth must have had a greater inheritance than this. In 1843, he owned the old family home in Garsdale, Swarthgill, as well as three other farms that had belonged to his grandfather, Birkrigg, Fawcetts, and Garsdale Hall. He did not retain these properties, for by 1859 they belonged to Sedbergh's doctor, Bryan Batty, and his wife and sister-in-law. Archives of the Sedbergh and District Historical Society. Francis Haygarth was educated at Harrow School and served in the army, where he attained the rank of colonel. He saw action at the Battle of the Alma in the Crimea. He seems to have inherited the longevity of the Haygarths, eventually dying in London in 1911, at the age of 91. Olive Haygarth, "Family History of John Haygarth."

It is clear that John Haygarth was motivated by his Christian beliefs. He was committed, as was his friend John Dawson, to the doctrines of the Anglican Church. Although so many of his friends—Thomas Percival, John Fothergill, John Aikin, and James Currie—were dissenters whose creeds he neither shared nor approved, they never allowed doctrinal differences to disturb their friendship. They were bound together by a common interest in science, the practice of medicine, and philanthropy. They were not, as some social historians have argued, interested in gaining power over their patients' bodies in the way that priests sought to dominate their minds. Haygarth seems to have had a particular gift for friendship, that "peculiar boon of heav'n" to use Johnson's phrase, and he never lost a friend except to the Almighty. Devoted as he was to the welfare of mankind, he is to be remembered particularly for his work on the prevention of infectious fevers, but also for his concern with education and the savings banks movement. It may not be immodest to place him, together with many others less well known, alongside the great pioneering philanthropists of his time, such as John Howard, William Wilberforce, and Elizabeth Fry. They were all individualists, pursuing their ends in different ways. But they shared the same aspiration: They strove to leave the world a better place than when they entered it.

Index